DISEASES

OF THE

SKIN

THEIR CONSTITUTIONAL NATURE AND HOMEOPATHIC CURE

J. COMPTON BURNETT, M.D.

B. JAIN PUBLISHERS (P) LTD.

USA — EUROPE — INDIA

DISEASE OF THE SKIN – THEIR CONSTITUTIONAL NATURE AND HOMEOPATHIC CURE

7th Impression: 2013

Published by Kuldeep Jain for

B. JAIN PUBLISHERS (P) LTD.
1921/10, Chuna Mandi, Paharganj, New Delhi 110 055 (INDIA)
Tel.: +91-11-4567 1000   Fax: +91-11-4567 1010
Email: info@bjain.com   Website: **www.bjain.com**

Printed in India by
J.J. Offset Printers

ISBN: 978-81-319-0042-0

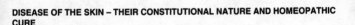

PREFACE TO THIRD EDITION.

FOR this third edition, I have added PART THIRD, dealing with the *cure of alopecia areata by constitutional remedies* without any local applications whatever. And it seems to me that if the disease can be cured by the exhibition of constitutional remedies in purely dynamic dose, the said disease must itself be of a constitutional quality, as the nature of the curative means indicates the nature of the malady.

J. COMPTON BURNETT.

86, WIMPOLE STREET, CAVENDISH SQUARE,
LONDON, W.,
Christmas 1897.

PREFACE TO SECOND EDITION.

THIS present edition I have very considerably enlarged by adding PART
SECOND, consisting more particularly of
Cases illustrating the constitutional Cure of
Diseases of the skin, and this has necessi-
tated an alteration in the title of the work.
Almost every day brings me evidence con-
firmatory of my views of the nature of constitutional skin diseases, and I am increas-
ingly impressed with the dire results that
accure to those sufferers therefrom whose
cutaneous manifestations have been got rid
of by lotions and ointments.

LONDON, W.

Midsummer 1893.

PREFACE TO FIRST EDITION.

IN the following pages I take largely the clinical standpoint, and consider the Diseases of the Skin constitutionally. The treatment of skin diseases as merely local affairs concerning the skin only, as is now current with *nearly* all medical men of all schools and all the world over, is, in my opinion, nothing less than a crime against humanity, and eminently characteristic of the cultured shallowness of the medical profession of to-day.

In 'these days of "scopes and meters," *thinking*, in the profession, is well-nigh dead. One sees no end of percussing and auscultating : the faintest murmurs, sounds, tinkles, *râles* and *bruits* are well known and learnedly discoursed of, but what of the *curing* ? what of the *real* ætiology of the Consumptive process itself ? Bacilli. Yes, but what went on before bacillary life became possible ? and how are the bacilli to thrive unless the soil be, for them, of the right kind ?

I do not maintain that there is no such a thing as a skin disease of a purely local nature, such as common phtheiriasis and other parasitic dirt-diseases that impinge upon the skin, but, speaking generally, I do maintain the following points :—

1. That the skin is a very important living ORGAN of the body.

2. That it stands in intimate, though ill-understood, relationship to *all* the internal organs and parts.

3. That its healthiness is conditioned by the general healthiness of the organism —*i. e.*, a healthy skin on an unhealthy body is inconceivable.

4. That, speaking generally, its unhealthiness—its diseases—come from within,

sometimes even when they initially impinge upon it from without.

5. That being *biologically within* the organism, being *fed from within*, having its *life from within*, having its *health from within*, and having its *diseases from within*, it must also be treated medicinally *from within*.

6. That skin diseases are most commonly not merely organic, but at the same time organismic, or constitutional.

7. That the skin being an excretory organ, and being spread out all over the organism, is often made use of by Nature to keep the internal organs free from disease.

8. That as each portion of the skin corresponds vitally with some internal organ or part, so the skin disease is often merely the outward expression of internal disease.

9. That, in fine, the generally received *external* treatment of Diseases of the Skin, whether with lotions or ointments or whatsoever else, is demonstrably shallow in conception, wrong in theory, harmful in practice, and therefore inadvisable.

These points embody my views on Diseases of the skin ; they guide me in my practice, and I might call upon the dermatologists to refute them, did I not hold them to be absolutely irrefutable.

If disease of the body bubbles up, so to speak, into the skin like water from a spring, to treat this Disease in (of) the skin by washes and ointments, or other outward applications, is really *not* treating the *diseased state* at all, but *only preventing its peripheral* expression.

The skin does not live an independent life of itself—hung on, as it were, outside of us—but is of all our organs the most systemic ; but what can we expect from an age in which people think they get a beautiful healthy skin from soap, and sound teeth from tooth-powder ?

The bark of a tree is a very fair analogue of the skin, and when I one day asked my gardener why the bark of a certain apple tree was so knobby, rough, and unhealthy-looking, he replied, "The *roots* have got down on the clay, Sir."

So it is, I opine, when a person's skin becomes diseased. "The roots have got. down on the clay."

LONDON, *September, 1886.*

DISEASES OF THE SKIN.

PART I.

Angina Pectoris from Suppressed Skin Disease.

ONE Sunday morning, some ten years ago, a gentleman ushered his wife into my consulting-room because she had been taken with an attack of *angina pectoris* in the street, on her way to church. Though only a little over thirty years of age, if so much, she had been subject to these attacks of breast-pang for several years : they would take her suddenly in the street, nailing her, as it were, to the spot, and hence she no longer went out of doors alone, lest she should faint away or fall down dead, as was apprehended.

An examination of the heart revealed no organic lesion, or even functional derangement, and I could not quite see why a comparatively young lady should get such anginal attacks. She had been under able men for her *angina*, but it got no better, and no one could apparently understand it. I prescribed for her, and saw her subsequently at her home, to try and elucidate the matter. I let her tell me her whole health-story from her earliest childhood. She said she was getting to the end of her teens, and was preparing to come out, but she had some cracks in the bends of her arms that were very unsightly ; these cracks in her skin had troubled her from her earliest childhood. Erasmus Wilson was consulted ; he gave her an ointment which very soon cured her skin, and the patient came out socially, made a hit right off, and got married in due course. She had always felt very grateful to Erasmus Wilson for curing her arms, for otherwise, "How could I have appeared in short sleeves."

But there soon followed dyspepsia, flatulence, dyspnoea, and palpitation, and finally the before described attacks of *angina pectoris* threatened to wreck her life. Moreover, she had borne one dead child. As I have already said, there was no discoverable cardiac lesion, and from the lady's health-history I gathered that this cure of her skin (though to me the one important point) was of no casual importance.

I gave my opinion that her skin disease had never been *really* cured, only *driven in* by Wilson's ointment, and that her angina was in reality its internal expression or metastasis. No one believed it, however. I began to treat her antipsorically, and very soon—I think it was less than a month from the Sunday morning visit--the old cracks reappeared in the bends of the elbows, *and from that time on she had no further attacks of angina* at all, and thenceforth she bore living children.

Specific Enexanthematic Asthma.

Not long after the before-mentioned experience I was consulted by a Liverpool gentleman for asthma of a very severe type. He was somewhere near forty, and had the appearance of a very old man, partly from the habitual bent position, from his shortness or breath, and partly from loss of sleep and much physicking. About a third of his life was spent in these attacks of asthma. In listening to his life-history, I noticed that he dated his asthma to a cold caught during a child's disease with a cutaneous eruption, and also, judging from his subjective ·symptoms, I concluded that he was suffering from an enexanthema, an internal skin disease of a specific nature. I treated him nearly a year on this hypothesis, and he got a strange coppery condition of the skin, which peeled of almost all over his body, much of his hair falling out at the same time. He was forthwith free of his asthma, and never had it again during the two following years, at the end of which period I lost sight of him. His skin be-

came quite healthy, and his hair
grew again.

Asthma, Psoriasis, and En-
larged Liver.

A gentleman of thirty came under my care some years since, suffering from asthma, enlargement
of the liver, psoriasis, and eczema.
When his skin was very bad, his
breathing was well ; and conversely
if his skin got well, he was almost
sure to get an attack of asthma,
particularly in certain places. I
treated his liver and his skin for
many months—in fact, for nearly
three years. It is now nearly two
years since he had any attack of
asthma, and he is well of both skin
2

and liver, though sun and wind still affect his skin unduly.

Hydrocephalus, Eczema, Latent Vaccinosis.

In the early part of the year 1885 I was requested to see the only surviving child of a country clergyman, who had been given up by three medical men, as it had water on the brain. The child's head was of the usual hydrocephalic type ; he was alternately wakeful and delirious at night, and he talked nonsense by day at intervals. Their local doctors had taken a consultant's opinion, and they agreed that the boy was suffering from tuberculosis of the meninges with effusion, of which a little brother had previously died. The child's life-history was told to me, and I underlined the facts that he had had eczema, and had been twice *un*successfully vaccinated. After the *un*successful vaccinations (want of organismic reactionary power) the eczema almost disappeared, and very soon the present disease began. I treated the case thus causally *ex-hypothesi* ; a severe pustular eruption, and then patches of lepra and eczema appeared, and at the end of about six months' treatment I was able to discharge the little patient, cured of his water on the brain and of his skin diseases. I saw him the other day, and learned that he continues well and has grown a good deal,

Eczema Capitis Suppressed— Fatal Issue.

About nine years ago the wife of a staff-officer brought her bonny little baby to me : it had the milk-crusty scalp, so horrible to aesthetic mothers—in fact, it had *crusta lactea, or eczema captis.* The scalp appeared one solid crust of scabs, but the child seemed perfectly well and jolly. I prescribed for the child *constitutionally*, and forbade all local treatment. The lady's father, however, was a retired physician of repute, and he went to stay at the daughter's house. Seeing the grandchild's eczema, he told the mother to use an ointment to the scalp. She told her father of my warning not to put anything on the bad head, but the old gentleman over-ruled it, and prescribed *unguentum zinci,* which soon healed the eczema. Abut a fortnight later I was suddenly summoned by telegram to see the child : it had been taken with convulsions from effusion on the brain, and the local doctors were already nonplussed. I did my best to get the eczema back on the surface of the scalp, but totally failed ; the child died, and the grandfather sobbingly cried, "Oh ! that zinc ointment."

Double Cataract from Suppressed Eruption.

A middlesex grocer brought his bright little boy of six or seven to

me about two years since : the boy
had double cataract, and was quite
blind. Said the father to me : He
used to have an eruption on his
head, but that was cured by the
doctors at the —— Hospital for
Diseases of the Skin. And soon
after he was cured of his eruption
we noticed his sight was failing—
before that his sight was all right.

Eczema, Ophthalmia.

A lady of fifty came under my
care in October 1879. Two years
previously she had had eczema of
the vulva, with much nocturnal irritation. Dr. W. cured it with bran
water and vegetal diet. In August
1879 she got eczema behind the

right ear, when her physician gave her *Graphite* **3ˣ** and *Merc. sol.* **3ˣ** in alternation.

In September of the same year she went to A—, and there met a doctor, who gave her a saline draught, and an ointment containing zinc, lead, and mercury, to be applied at night.

This cured the eczema. She came to me for an inflammation of right eye, that came very soon after the eczema was cured. I explained to her that the ophthalmia and the eczema were really the same thing, and advised constitutional treatment, to which she consented. She *was worse at the sea-side,*

she was constipated, her skin was
dry, *salt* beef caused constipation
and faintness, and she was low-
spirited. *Natrum muriaticum 6*, trit.,
and other remedies, cured her
constitutionally, and she had not
had any return of skin disease or
ophthalmia, when her husband
called on me, on June 2nd, 1885, or
more than five years thereafter.

Ossified Heart from Suppressed Eczema.

In the year 1874, I was attending a country squire for eczema of
the whole body of a very bad
type,—in fact I never saw a worse
case. He could not undress without laying a sheet on the carpet, as
the quantity of dried scabs that fell

off was really considerable : after
undressing he was in the habit of
using the coal-shovel to shovel
them up. I treated him to the
best of my ability for a long time,
but in vain ; he grew rather
worse than better. I called in a
consultant of very great experience
and world-wide reputation, and we
treated the case together ; but the
eczema defied us, and so did the
patient too. He sent for me one
day, said he was sick of the weary,
weary "constitutional treatment" of
which I was always telling him. I
solemnly warned him against local
measures, such as baths and ointments, saying : "Remember this,
Mr.——, I acknowledge that I have
quite failed to cure your eczema

with my 'constitutional treatment,' at which it pleases you to poke fun, but *you yourself never enjoyed better health in your life*, although your eczema is indeed almost as bad as ever. You are disgusted with your foul disease, and you mean to be rid of its outward expression, come what may. I am sorry for you."

He went to an eminent special skin doctor, now deceased, and in a few months was cured of his eczema by means of ointments, washes, and mineral waters.

For four years I did not see him, and then he called to consult me *about difficulty of breathing* that had been slowly creeping on for several years,—in fact was first felt not long after his being cured by Mr. S. of eczema. I should have said that the patient in question told his skin doctor of my warnings anent his eczema, and this gentleman made light of it, declaring that it was my incompetence to cure that deserved attention, and used such language about me professionally that my patient would not allow my name to be mentioned in his house for nearly three years. Then his dyspnoea became a serious matter, and his physicians all failed to cure it, though they all declared that his lungs were sound. At last he found that an extra glass of champagne, a tiny incline, the gentlest game of croquet, all upset his breathing, and the doctors' skill failing, too, he went to the South of France, and to spas, and then to lung specialists, but all to no purpose—his breathing slowly and surely grew worse. Finally he came to me, "to please his wife." He seemed quite well to look at ; there was no trace of his former eczema on his skin ; his lungs were all right, but his heart was irregular in its action, and there was neither apex-beat nor radial pulse. No medicines did him any real or permanent good, though many well-chosen remedies relieved his various symptoms ; in fact, I cured all his symptoms over and over again, and then he died of his disease. We had a *post-mortem* examination of the body, and found ossification of the heart in about two-thirds of its extent, with osseous and quasi-osseous adhesions to the diaphragm, and shrinking of the liver.

No doubt, to my mind, about the genesis of the degeneration of the internal organs. When Nature was prevented from speaking as eczema by Mr. S.'s skin-gagging, she used the internal parts wherein to deposit the irritant material which produced inflammation and ossification of the most vital organ—the heart—rendering a continuation of its functions impossible. Such are the facts, and such my reading thereof.

In these pages I rely purposely on my own observations exclusively, but the following excerpt from the very orthodox *Record* is so consonant with my views, that I here interpolate it :—

Disappearance of Psoriasis and Trachoma after Erysipelas.

Striking instances of internal affections being cured by some outward, or other acute manifestation constantly recur in medical literature. A few years since I was reading in the *London Medical Record* (April 15, 1886, p. 155, *et seq.*), that—

"Dr. Porfiry G. Bazaroff, of Belyi Klutch, records (*Proceedings of the Caucasian Medical Society*, No. 18, 1885, p. 433) the case of a highly scrofulous soldier, aged 22, who was admitted with general psoriasis vulgaris of two years' duration, severe trachoma of long standing on both sides, and enlargement of the cervical and submaxillary glands. The treatment failing to relieve any of the patient's extremely obstinate and troublesome affections, the regimental surgeons resolved upon placing him on the roll of 'unfit for service.' About that time, however, the patient was suddenly attacked by erysipelas of the face and head. There was nothing peculiar either in the course or in the treatment of the disease. The erysipelas disappeared

in seven days, and with it the
trachoma, the glandular swellings
and psoriasis (first of the face, then
—after two hot baths—of the re-
maining parts) also disappeared,
leaving no trace. 'In fact, in a
week an "unfit" became quite a
healthy man,' the author adds. Dr.
Bazaroff mentions, also, a rather
obscure case of a young soldier,
who had suffered from daily and
nightly in-continence of urine, of
two months' duration, and who got
rid of the symptoms after an attack
of erysipelas of the face and head.
In another patient, a boy, aged 22
months, with congenital hydroce-
phalus of the progressive kind, a
mild attack of scarlatina was followed by a steady diminution in the

bulk of the head (in a month the large circumference lessened a centimetre, the minor 3), an improvement in his general state, &c. Two months later, however, the child died from general convulsions. [Dr. M. Tumpovsky recently published a case of disappearance of ascites from erysipelas (see the *London Medical Record*, May, 1885, p. 19,) Dr. K. Koltchevsky saw a case of trachoma cured by erysipelas (*Ib.*, July, p. 296). Dr. Mishtolt's patient was cured by the same disease from sarcoma (*Ib.*, January, 1884, p. 11). In the *Vratch*, Nos. 38—41, 1882, Dr. F. J. Pasternatzky, of Professor J. T. Tchudnovskys clinic, details two cases of the disappearance of hepatic ascites under the influence of typhus fever, and a case of renal dropsy cured by relapsing fever. In the *St. Petersburg Med. Wochensch.*, No. 43, 1883, Dr. Schmidt published a case where erysipelas of the chest had caused a rapid disappearance of an enormous pleuritic exudation —*Rep.*]"

All this surely proves that topic disease is not local, but *organic and organismic.*

Eczema with Internal Metastatic Symptoms.

A few years since—May, 1886 —I met with a very striking example of the intimate connection that exists between a skin affliction and internal symptoms. I had seen the lady in town and prescribed for her on April 13th, 1886, and I received the following letter, subsequently. I give it just as I received it, and will let it tell its own simple though instructive tale—

"A few days after I came to see you I was very unwell—at the usual time—which commenced four days too soon, and lasted nine days. On the fourth day, Sunday, April 18th, I was taken at 5 A. M. with fainting, &c., as before ; took brandy just in time to prevent going quite off. This was followed by sickness, alternate heat and chill, and I was unable to take any food without causing sickness ; I

was so ill that my brother became
anxious, and sent for the nearest
homoeopathic doctor. The sickness
continued frequently until he arrived
about I. P. M. I was very weak and
in my room for some days.

"During this time the eruption
on hands and face disappeared,
and the cracks healed, but as soon
as I recovered it broke out again
and was worse than ever on my
face, large patches of spots conti-
nually running, with heat and
irritation. Both face and hands
were much swollen, and the eruption extended to wrists and neck—
right side of neck below the ear
being swollen and tender.

"After a few days the fingers and backs of hand became very badly cracked; for ten days I could scarcely use my hands, and they are still very sore ; there is less tendency to heal than usual, and considerable irritation ; the joints of fingers are also swollen."

This lady had previously had catalepsy on various occasions, and she consulted me for the neurosis principally.

Eruption on Scalp—Cataract.

The following case is very instructive, as showing the nature of a skin affection of the head (scalp), and its power of expressing itself in the lens if compelled to retire from the outer integument.

Towards the end of the year 1880, a boy of four was brought to me from the South of England. His sight was good until he was about two years old, when he had incipient cataract in the right eye, then in the left one, and at the age of three he was blind.

I elicited the following noteworthy anamnestic point : He used to have great irritation of the skin ever since he was a few months old ; when between eight and nine months old he was treated for it with "sulphur ointment, a lotion, and medicines."

After the first medicine which I ordered him an eruption came on his skin, and more particularly on the scalp, and he began to see ! His mother reported that he altered in his gait, for whereas he formerly looked straight out before him fixedly at the light, now he bends forward. He further astonished his parents by remarking that there was a certain colour in the painted ceiling, pale green. There was also slight but evident change in the opaque lenses themselves.

Now, although I had given to the parents, as my opinion, that the cataract was a direct consequence of the cured (suppressed) skin affection from which the child had suffered, still, no sooner did my medicine begin to bring back the eruption to the scalp than the mother forthwith applied some zinc ointment she had in the house! The zinc ointment did its work very promptly and effectually; the eruption disappeared, and so did the returning vision,—*i. e.*, the boy went quite blind again, and remained so. He also began to talk, laugh, and cry in his sleep again as he had previously done.

The further course of this case showed most conclusively that the opacity of the lenses, and the scalp eruption, stood in causal nexus,—that is to say, they had a common cause. Orthodox medicine *cured* the eruption with ointment, then came the cataract, which is again *cured* by operation. Truly, we live in an age of wisdom and enlightenment.

Vaccinal Dermatitis.

Although I hold that vaccination, in due:dose, protects, on the homoeoprophylactic principle, from small-pox, still it is nevertheless a fruitful source of skin diseases. I may be allowed to transcribe a few cases from: my little treatise, entitled "Vaccinosis and its Cure by Thuja, with Remarks on Homoeoprophylaxis" (London and New York, 1884), which illustrate this point, viz. :—

Pustular Eruption.

Mr. J—, a hale-looking, middle-aged London merchant, came under my observation on November 3rd, 1881. Said he, "I am not a homoeopath, but twenty years ago I had eczema, and the allopaths could not touch it, so I went to a homoeopathic doctor, and he cured me." And he went on to say that he believed in homoeopathy for skin diseases. On the left leg he had a pustular eruption, due, he believed, to a bruise. He had also eczema of the ear, and he volunteered the information that ever since his second vaccination he had been subject to eczema. The eczema of twenty years ago was soon after the re-vaccination.

℞ *Thujæ Occidentalis 30.* Four three-drop powders to the two dozen. To take one, dry on the tongue, three times a day.

He came in a week nearly well ; the pustules had at once begun to wither.

The *Thuja* was repeated, but in less frequent doses, and the patient subsequently sent word by his brother to say that his skin was well, and he himself too busy to show himself as he had promised.

Pustular Eruptions.

Miss ——, aet. 18, was re-vaccinated in july, 1881, at her parents' country residence, thirty miles from

London, by the local surgeon, with "lymph" direct from the calf. The operation was very successful, and she had a very "fine" arm. But as the "arm" was just at its greatest perfection she got an eruption on her chin, covering its whole extent and involving the lower lip. The thing was very unsightly, and had a singularly ugly, repulsive aspect. The gentleman who had done the re-vaccination was of opinion that Miss —— had got some of the vaccine virus on to her finger-nails and inoculated herself by scratching. The sequel, however, showed that the chin manifestation was from within. The surgeon had ordered applications, two of which were vaseline and zinc ointment, but the

eruption on the chin was not to be
got rid of. The young lady had to
wear a dense veil to hide her face
when driving out. She was brought
to London for my advice, and I
gave *Thuja 30*. In a fortnight she
was out and about, and only some
diffused redness of the skin remained, but no scar or thickened
skin. Now, it might be objected to
this case that the *Thuja* had nothing to do with the disappearance
of the eruption, because it was just
the history of the disease : it ran
through its natural course and died.
I thought that to myself at the time
of prescribing it ; but against this
was the fact that the arm had healed
already, and it had passed the
natural course of vaccinia by at

least a fortnight when I first prescribed the *Thuja*. But to have a
test, I gave her brother, who also
had a somewhat similar pustular
eruption (and who had been re-vaccinated at the same time), but more
spare, and instead of being on the
chin, it was around the left nostril,
I say, to have a test, I gave this
brother of Miss———— *Antimonium
tart.*, which is also, as every one
knows, apparently homoeopathic to
such a pustular eruption.

This is the brother of Miss————
(*observ. iv.*)

The two eruptions were similar,
though the boy's was comparatively
trivial, and of the same age, and
from the same cause, *i. e.*, from the

vaccine virus. The patients went into the country, and in two or three weeks' time the mother wrote that the young lady was quite well: "the medicine soon put the right," was her expression, but the boy had "a bad cold in his head; nose-bleed; left side of nose swelled and red; two little spots of matter, the size of a large pin's head, at the edge of the nostril, and below it, having something the look of——'s chin; his arm is also not well, and he has had four little pocks about the vaccination marks." I sent *Thuja* **30**, and he was reported well in ten days.

If any one can account for the cure of these two cases independ-

ently of the *Thuja*, his ingenuity is
greater than mine. That they were
causally connected with the re-vaccination admits of no doubt whatever.

Hairless Patches on Chin.

Mr. ——, a London merchant,
came under my care on July 27th,
1882, to be treated for same
roundish hairless patches on either
side of his chin, which began four
months ago. The larger patch on
the right side was about the size
of a florin. Had also an old hordeolum on his right lower eyelid.

Has been twice vaccinated; the
second time, twelve years ago, did
not "take."

℞. *Thuja Occidentalis* *30* (4 in 24). To take one, dry on the tongue, at bedtime.

Sept. 7th.—The bald patches are smaller, the one on the left side nearly gone. Has, apparently, a very bad coryza—(?) organismic reaction.

Rep.

Oct. 17th.—The bald patches are gone ; the old hordeolum also gone.

The closely-shaven beard is now uniform, the previously-existing white bald patches being completely covered with hair.

I give this as an interesting cure by *Thuja*, but I am not very sure that the disease was really due to vaccinosis, because of other points

in his clinical history. Still it might
have been so, as the hair is very
powerfully influenced by the vaccine poisoning. Thus Kunkel observed both a very weak growth of
hair and an excessive growth, especially in wrong places, as effects,
he believed, of vaccination. Therefore, let it stand as a doubtful case
of vaccinosis for what it may be
worth,—but there can hardly be
any reasonable doubt as to the cure
of the case by *Thuja*.

Here it might not be amiss to
observe casually 'that the presence
of sties on the eyelids is often, in
my opinion, a symptom of vacciono-,
sis. This case is not without practical importance, inasmuch as ho-

diernal medicine hands over a sty
to the chirurgeon's art ; and all the
time, poor old dame, weens herself
so very much superior to scientific
therapeutics usually called homoeopathy. The conceit of the ortho-
doxly ignorant is truly sickening.

Acne of Face and Nose, and Nasal Dermatitis.

A young lady, about twenty years
of age, was brought by her mother
to me on October 28th, 1882.
Patient had a very red pimply nose,
not like the red nose of the elderly
bibber, or like that due to dyspepsia
or to tight-lacing, but a pimply,
scaly nasal dermatitis, which ex-

tended from the cutaneous covering of the nose to that of the cheeks, but appearing more as facial acne. The nasal dermatitis was, roughly, in the form of a saddle. Of course this state of things in an otherwise pretty girl of twenty was painfully and humiliatingly unpleasant to her and to her friends,—in fact, it was likely to mar her future prospects very materially, more especially as it had already existed for six years and was making no signs of departing. She also complained of obstinate constipation. The pimples of the nose and face used to get little white mattery heads. In trying to trace the skin-affection back to its real origin I ascertained that the patient was re-vaccinated six years ago, but she could not remember whether the nose was previously affected or not. This re-vaccination was unsuccessful, *i.e.*, it did *not* "take."

℞ *Thuja Occidentalis 30.*

November 30th.— Pimples of face decidedly better. Nose less red. Constipation no better.

℞ *Thuja Occidentalis 100.*

January 3rd, 1883.—The face is free ! Her mother gratefully exclaims, "She is wonderfully better." I ask the young lady which powders did her *most good* , she says, "The *last.*" The skin of the nose is normal, but the constipation is no better, and for this she remains under treatment.

That *Thuja* cured this case is incontrovertible ; but that it was a case of vaccinosis is not quite so certain, though it is far from improbable. The re-vaccination and inflammation of the skin of the nose were referred both to six years ago when she was in Switzerland at school ; but patient could not remember which was first—the bad nose or the vaccination.

Diseased Finger-nails.

On December 22nd, 1882, a young lady of twenty-six came under my care for an ugly state of the nails of her fingers. Naturally a lady of her age would not be indifferent to the state of her nails.

These nails are indented rather deeply, ane in addition to these indentations there are black patches on the under surfaces of the nails, reaching into the quick. Very slight leucorrhoea occasionally. She had chicken-pox as a child of eleven. On her shoulders there is an eruption of roundish patches forming mattery heads. Has been vaccinated three different times; the last time two years ago, and the nails have become diseased *since* this last vaccination. The black patches have existed these eighteen months.

Looking upon this-diseased condition of the nails as evidence of chronic vaccinosis, I ordered her *Thuja 30* (one in 6).

March 19th, 1883.—Has continued the *Thuja 30* for just about three months, with the result that within a fortnight from commencing with it the black patches under the nails began to disappear, and there is now no trace of them. The indentations are notably better. The eruption on the back has not been modified, and for this she remains under treatment ; but I thought this much of a case of nail disease would be of some interest, and the more so as it is not easy to demonstrate drug-action on nail growth at all.

The foregoing cases sufficiently exemplify the causal nexus existing, as I believe, between vaccination and diseases of the skin. However, by no means must be attributed all skin affection, following closely or remotely in the wake of vaccination, to the pathogenetic effect of the vaccine virus itself ; it *does* cause numerous skin diseases without a doubt, but it also, and frequently, *rouses latent disease* for which anti-vaccinial treatment will, of course, not suffice.

Ringworm of Scalp—Cataract.

At the beginning of 1883 a boy of six was brought to me, from Yorkshire, with opacities of both lenses. The failing of his sight was first noticed in 1881. Had been under an oculist of repute, who had given some drops to be

put into the eyes, but these drops
could not be used after the first
instillation, as they "made the
child like a dead'un for days."
Has been delicate all his life, and
notably worse since the measles in
the summer of 1880.

Had ringworm of the scalp in
the summer of 1879, which was
cured by internal (probably tonic)
and external treatment. The father
says he is "wick," which he explains means *lively*. After four
months of Sulphur 30, and then of
the 200th, this report came—"My
boy is still improving with his eyes
slowly , they have not that large,
glaring appearance , look more
natural, and he has not been

excited in his sleep ; I think his head is cooler."

A little later I received a letter to say that the boy had "ringworm on his scalp again !" That was the last I heard of him.

The connection of cataract and various skin affections has long been noticed and written about by numerous authors, but the doctrine is not accepted by many. On this point I take the liberty of referring to my treatise on Cataract,∗ which, through the kindness of my learned friend, Dr. Goullon, of Weimar, has lately been translated into German. From it I quote the following, bearing thereon (pp. 47, 48).

∗ "Curability of Cataract with Medicines." London and New York, 1880.

Scabies—Cataract—Furuncles.

Young man, aet. 20, had had the itch one year and a half ago, of which he got rid by internal and external use of medicines. Later, he had an attack of intermittent fever, which he cured with pepper and whisky. A short time since he discovered that he could not see with his left eye. The eye had a dead look ; pupil was enlarged and immovable ; in the middle of the lens there was an opacity, as if it had been punctured by a needle ; the lids and conjunctiva were somewhat reddened. On holding the hand quite near to the eye he could dimly discern the fingers. August 2, *Sulphur 6* ; August 9, SEVERAL

PIMPLES ON THE FACE AND ARMS
Sight better. *Sulph.* *6*, which was
repeated on the 19th, 26th, and
29th of August, and on the 3rd
and 23rd of September. THERE
APPEARED A NUMBER OF FURUNC-
LES ON THE ARMS ; the eye looks
natural again, and he sees as well
as ever before.— (Fr. Emmerich,
"Arch." XIV., iii, p. 105. In Raue.)

And then (pp. 7-78)—

Dr. Bernard gives an epitome
of fifteen cases from Ruckert's
Klinische Erfahrungen.

I will only give the fifteenth at
this place.

Crusta Lactea.

The fifteenth is this : *Crusta lactea*
disappears and cataract supervenes,

which latter is cured with *Spirit
Sulph.* (*Autore*, Schoenfeld).

Dr. Bernard also notes that in
several of the cases habitual perspirations re-appear, or a cutaneous
eruption either appears or re-ap-
pears.

Need we any further proof that
cataract is a *cutaneous* affection ?

Tetters.

Dr. Becker treated a carpenter
who had been affected for some
time with tetters about the face,
which disappeared after a while
without his taking any medicine,
but his sight became impaired,
everything appeared in a place
different from its real position, so

that he was unable to use his tools properly.

The pupils presented a misty, smoky appearance, as in the forming stage of cataract. He received *Sp. Sulph.*, ten drops three times a day ; *the old eruption re-appeared*, and he now saw everything in the right position, but otherwise his sight was not improved.

Then on March 22nd, *Aq. Silic.* was administered in doses of seven drops daily, and this was followed by a great improvement in his sight. He perspired easily, and had much perspiration about the feet. Deposit in urine like lime.

July.—A rheumatic inflammation of the foot set in.

Suppressed Perspiration of Feet.

The same gentleman treated a lady whose feet generally perspired freely and then became very dry, and thereafter she noticed that her sight became affected in such a manner that everything she looked at appeared to be enveloped in a cloud ; she could only read large print.

Aq. Silic. was administered in doses of ten drops twice a day. *The accustomed perspiration of the feet returned again* in about a month. Her eyesight became much better. Two months latter, at the time of menstruation, her eyes became worse again, and she then took twenty drops *Ac. Silic.* three times a day, after which she improved very much, could read better, and continued taking the same remedy

Scabies—Ague.

(Pp. 98, 99, 100)—

M., aged 20, tinsmith by trade, was affected a year and a half ago with the worst kind of itch, and subsequently with fever and ague. Sometimes he had tearing pains in the left eye, and some itching of the skin, to which he paid very little attention; suddenly he noticed, however, that he had become completely blind in the left eye.

Symptoms.—A staring look of the left eye ; pupil dilated and immovable ; in the centre of the lens

there was slight opacity ; his sight
was almost extinguished.

Treatment.—*August 2.*—*Sulph. 6* ;
from August 9th to September
23rd, six doses of the same.

Six days after the first dose, *many
pustules appeared on the face and
arms ;* in the meanwhile his eyesight improved so much that he
was enabled to distinguish large
letters. From September 13th to
September 23rd, *furuncles on the
arm made their appearance ;* after
that the skin became clear again,
and the affected eye was as useful
as it had ever been before,—
("Arch." XIV., v., p. 105. Emmerich.)

Of the connection of the skin and the lens embryologically and pathologically I will say no more, merely referring those interested in the subject for further information to "Curability of Cataract."

The "Sternal Patch".

One often meets with liver affections connected with cutaneous manifestations.

I would like particularly to refer to a patch of eruption on the skin covering the lower part of the sternum, which I have several times found co-exist with heart disease and swelling of the left lobe of the liver. In my case-takings I call it in the "sternal patch."

I have four such cases in my mind at this moment. The first I will narrate is that of a mayor of a large town in the north :—He had a patch of brownish lichen on the sternal portion of thorax, of the size of a woman's palm ; with it were associated an enlarged liver and a cardiac affection, evidenced by palpitation, systolic murmur, and general uneasiness. He came to town to see me at odd intervals for about two years, and was then discharged cured. I treated him antipsorically and organopathically, the most notable benefit being derived from *Carduus Mariœ* in five drop doses of the strong tincture given three times a day.

The second, I remember, was a Manchester merchant, with the same kind of cutaneous patch on the sternum, and very notable heart trouble, with arcus senilis as a concomitant. Here the case and comfort brought by the *Carduus Mariæ* were very striking. Under date of January 31st, 1883, I find in my case-book these words of the enthusiastic patient,—"It had a most marvellous effect ; soon made me right ; the patch went away in a fortnight ; had had it for years."

This gentleman has remained under my care, calling upon me at odd times when in town, and during the past two years has

had, besides the strong tincture
of *Carduus, Bellis perennis 1,
Aurum metallicum 4, Vanadium
6,* and *Acidum oxalicum 3^x*, and
some other remedies, and I consider him vastly improved, and
his life—speaking commercially—
worth 40 per cent. more than
previously.

The third case was that of a
New York merchant, who suffered
from liver, and had come over to
Europe to consult a physician, as
he seemed to get no better from
the treatment of his New York
advisers. I found his liver very
much enlarged, and also the
before-mentioned sternal patch of
skin disease. I gave him *Carduus*

in like dose to the foregoing, and he came in a week declaring himself quite well. I advised him to remain awhile under observation, to see if the cure proved permanent, but he hurried out of my room in great glee, and I never saw him again.

The fourth case in which I found the sternal patch and enlarged liver, giddiness, and palpitations of the heart, was that of a London lawyer. Here the liver got well, and the heart too, together with the giddiness, but it needed a course of antipsoric treatment to finish the cure of the patch of diseased skin. I might say the same of a fifth case,—an officer in

the Royal Navy, where this patch
co-exists with hypertrophied liver,
and in which the affair has a
specific air about it, probably in-
herited

Sarcognomy.

I foretell that, in the future,
when the relations of the various
cutaneous regions will be recognised as constituting the very base
of medical and medicinal diagnosis,
this *sternal patch* will be under-
stood to indicate "liver and heart."

Chin and Throat Affections.

At the commencement of 1873
a young lady came from a distance

to consult me in regard to her throat. She told me she had originally relaxed sore throat, and went to Mr. ——, who cauterized it a good many times, and she used gargles and other local means on his advice. Her throat became better, but she then got a series of quinsies. Then came recommendations of changes of air and tonics. She had thereafter nothing to complain of in her throat, but her chin had become the seat of some nasty spots. For these she returned to the same gentleman, who cured the chin with ointment. After her chin got well her throat again troubled her. Renewed cauterizings ; throat again cured. Then the face and chin were covered with spots and pimples afresh. So she went on for six years under the most many-sided surgeon of the day, who writes so very philosophically about the pedigree of disease, but who treats his patients generally locally all the same, absolutely unmindful of the twaddling dictum about "gleams of a fruitful suggestion." Well, as this young lady's chin and throat persisted in playing hide and seek, she felt constrained to try something else. I went into the case carefully, and found that the real *seat* of the constitutional disturbances giving rise to the symptoms in the throat and on the chin was neither in the throat nor in the chin, but in the *ovaries*, and so, of course, the silly treating of the throat and chin had led to nothing.

The Absurdity of Specialism.

Probably it would not be easy to obtain a more striking example of the absurdity and futility of ordinary local treatment usual with most of the so-called specialists than this :—

Miss Nora———, twenty-four years of age, was brought to me in June 1885, that I might give my *opinion* of her case. My treatment was not sought at that time. Twelve years previously she had scarlet fever, and following thereon, measles. Ever since then she has been deaf. She has been subject to hay fever these twelve years, and also bronchitis. Her father has hay fever, and also : one of her brothers. She is also subject to a very severe form of nettle-rash ; at her menstruation she suffers "excruciating agony," and the discharge is very profuse and very clotted ; very bad leucorrhoea.

The treatment she had was at first that of their ordinary (homoeopathic) family physician, who, failing to relieve the dysmenorrhoea, took her to a gynaecologist of great reputation, who performed an operation, but it did no good at all. She then was treated by the family doctor for her bronchitis. Then, she was sent away for her health for varying periods and to various places.

Now she is actually under two specialists; one treats the ear, and the other is treating her hay fever. In addition to these two learned brethren, her mother is also treating her "nettle-rash" with domestic homoeopathy.

With all this local tinkering and pottering and domestic messing, she is no better. No one has attempted to take a view of her entire economy as a living unity. Is it any wonder that all these fruitless measures have made the poor girl almost bewildered?

Relationship of Skin Affections to Internal Organs.

As illustrating the *general* nature of skin affections, and their intimate relationship with other organs and parts, I will narrate a part of the history of a lady of rank, now forty odd years of age.

Originally, some fifteen or more years ago, she had badly ulcerated legs, and her local surgeon cured them quickly with an ointment. Soon after this cure—of which both patient and doctor were very proud—she had ulcers on the eyes, which a late eminent oculist cauterized, without being able to get rid of them ; then a very noted

London physician saw her, and said he thought the ulcers on the eyes were due to the too rapid cure of the ulcerated skin of the legs, and ordered her to use vinegar compresses over her shins, with the object of inducing fresh ulcers ; but, *at the same time*, he ordered her to use golden ointment to the eye ulcers,—which golden salve forthwith cured them. The vinegar compresses produced an eruption on the legs, as they will on most people.

How this unctuous physician could give an opinion that the eye affection arose from the quasi-cured leg ulcers, and then forthwith order an ointment to cure the eye ulcers

on precisely the same lines, might
at first sight seem strange, only
one knows of him that he mistakes
a jumble of second-hand clinical
tips for laws of therapeutics.

Presently the poor patient
found that getting rid of corneal
and conjunctival ulcers with golden
ointment was anything but a cure
of the disease essentially, for the
next step of the progress of the
disease was *in* the eye, *not on* it. The
inside of the eye not lending itself
to unctuous handling, it was sought
out with the—knife ! The operation
had to be repeated several times.
Well, it's a long, weary, story, and
patient is nearly blind, and almost
eyeless these several years.

I was listening to this history two days ago, and the poor lady exclaimed, "Ah ! if I had but never used that golden ointment."

Eczema—Enlarged Ovary—Chronic Oophoritis.

It is about two years since a lady of forty came from a distance to see me ; she was an invalid, and had not had a month of good health for many years. I found her suffering from chronic oophoritis of the right side, which recrudesced every month at the menstrual time, and which was often accompanied by circumscribed peritonitis. The ovary was enlarged to about the size of an orange, was very tender,

and was clearly attached by post-
inflammatory adhesions to the
peritoneum. The dysmenorrhoea
was very terrible, and the periodical peritonitis was quite an
illness. She had leucorrhoea, and
her visage told the tale of great
and repeated sufferings. Treatment has quite cured her, and she
now leads an active, useful life; but
that is not the point I wish to dwell
upon, but rather upon its origin.

I found from her history that
she used to suffer from eczema ;
she went to Erasmus Wilson, who
prescribed "zinc ointment and
other things," and quickly cured
it (the eczema). Patient herself
denied "ever having had anything

the matter with her skin ;" it was her relations who told me of the old eczema.

People have certain preconceived ideas of diseases : if they know you are suffering from "liver," they smile ; if you have anything wrong with your brain, rendering you insane or vicious, they are afraid of you and lock you up in an asylum ; if you have anything wrong with your skin, they shun and despise you, little weening that the same or a like morbid essentiality may be at the bottom of them all. And hence, when questioned about their "skin." people not infrequently stop short of all the truth.

Constitutional Nature of Lupus.

It is very curious that even where some eminent and thoughtful dermatologists admit the constitutional nature of a given skin disease, they still adhere to the *local* treatment. For instance, it is now thought and taught by some advanced men that lupus is a tuberculous disease of a bacillary nature.

As giving the latest views on the pathology of lupus—the most terrible of all skin diseases—I should like to quote freely from Dr. Walter G. Smith's paper in the February (1885) number of the "Dublin Journal of Medical Science,"

Professor Smith says :—

"Turning now to the pathology of lupus, we find two chief views prevailing as to its aetiology—

"I. What may be termed the Anglo-French school,—*i. e.*, that lupus has a constitutional foundation, and is allied especially to scrofula.

"Mr. Jonathan Hutchinson seeks, with Auspitz, to widen the signification of lupus, and contends for a clinical 'lupus family' of affections. He regards lupus on the whole 'as a sort of cross produced by tendencies at once to scrofula and cancer, while it receives many modifications, from peculiarities in

the patient's skin and his morbid
tendenceis, in one or the other di-
rection'. It is interesting to note
that a similar view was put forward
as novel at the time by Dr. James
Houghton, fifty years ago :—'Were
we called on to declare our opinion
of the essential character of lupus,
we should say that it is an interme-
diate pathological state between
cancer and scrofula, partaking somewhat of the nature of both, but
constituting a state in which, by
the blending of these two diseases,
many of their peculiar characteris-
tics are lost.'

"2. The Vienna school, as re-
presented by Kaposi.—that lupus is
an exclusivly local affection, and

hence constitutional treatment is rejected as useless. But notwithstanding Kaposi and the arguments he adduces, converging evidence has been accumulating in favor of the doctrine that lupus is a branch of the tuberculous stock ; or in other words, that lupus will find its true place among the chronic infective diseases of the skin,—*i. e.*, those dependent upon the action of an organised virus capable of reproducing itself in the body (*e.g.*, lepra, syphilis, and tuberculosis).

"The following remarks refer particularly to lupus vulgaris, for the nature of lupus erythematosus is still a matter of controversy, and Veiel places it among the superficial inflammations of the skin along with eczema and impetigo.

"The question, then, is this—Syphilis has a specific virus, likewise leprosy and tuberculosis ; is it so with lupus ?

"Ziegler, while he places lupus among the infective granulomata, admits that 'the exciting cause of lupus is unknown.' Similarly Hyde—'The causes of lupus vulgaris are absolutely unknown ;' and Neisser, in his admirable article, to which I am largely indebted, and in which he upholds on general pathological grounds the tuberculous nature of lupus, says :—'But I cannot yet adduce the exact proof of this connection, since neither I nor others have hitherto succeeded in demonstrating with certainty the bacilli of tuberculosis in lupous material.' He presently adds that he holds the forthcoming proof to be only a question of time.

"The question may be conveniently studied from three points of view—viz., clinical, histological, and experimental.

"1. *Clinical Aspects.*—Upon this point suffice it to say that while Kaposi and his followers are unable to see any connection with scrofula or tubercle, and even ridicule the proposition, they have arrayed against them the testimony of numerous skilled observers in England, France, and Germany, who recognize the points of resemblance, and note the frequent coincidence of cheesy affections of the glands, bones, and joints with lupus. I cannot give statistics from my own cases, but certainly the association of lupus with scrofulous glands is sufficiently common here, and with Fagge and others, I have witnessed the development of lupus secondary to suppurative strumous inflammation.

"Now, since the fundamental unity of scrofulosis and tuberculosis has been established both on clinical and experimental grounds, if it can be shown that an intimate relation exists between lupus and scrofula, an argument will be furnished for bringing lupus into the tuberculous family. M. Besnier, one of the foremost French dermatologists, insists upon the connection between lupus and tuberculosis. In June and July 1883, among 38 patients under his care for lupus in St. Louis, 8 presented well-marked physical signs of phthisis. Dr. Tilbury Fox states that lupus, in many cases, occurs in phthisical subjects; and Mr. Hutchinson has pointed out that phthisis is not unfrequently observed in the families of those suffering from lupus.

"It is quite true that lupus is rarely observed in several members of the same family (Fagge), that it is seldom found in combination

with general tuberculosis, and that
we have no evidence of hereditary
or of direct transmission in the
human subject.

"2. *Histological*.—Careful investigations have shown that no essential difference can be established
between a caseating miliary tubercle and a lupous nodule, which
sometimes exhibits 'the exact appearance of tubercles (Ziegler). The
pathological processes in each are
the same in kind, but differ in
degree. Thus in lupus it is less
acute and less intense, and hence
we get slower development of
the inflammatory granuloma with
a richer development of vessels,
and consequently a more gradual

destruction towards the centre, with peripheral healing and formation of spindle cell-tissue,—*i. e.*, cicatrix (Neisser). But the decisive proof—the demonstration of tubercle-bacilli in lupus material—remained to be given, and it was not long before Neisser's prophecy was fulfilled Dr. Robert Koch, following up Friedlander's anatomical investigations, examined seven cases of lupus of unimpeachable diagnosis.

"In 4 cases he excised parts of the skin. In 3 cases he examined scrapings only of the lupous tissue.

"For direct microscopic investigation he used only the excised bits of skin. The tubercle-bacilli were found sparsely in each of the

4 cases, and only in the interior of
the giant-cells. The tubercle-bacilli
in lupous tissue are so isolated that
in 2 cases the bacilli were not found
until in the one case 27 sections,
and in the other 43 sections had
been made. Yet it repeatedly
happened that when in a number
of sections not a single bacillus
appeared, sections taken close by
exhibited one to three bacilli.
Koch never found more than one
bacillus in giant-cell.

"According to Unna, the bacilli are observable in quantity by
partially digested hardened speci-
mens, and examining the precipitate
that falls down. Demme, Pfeiffer,
and Doutrelepont had published

records of the occurrence of tubercle-bacilli in lupous skin, and in the tubercles of animals inoculated with lupus. But Koch states that his experiments were finished for some months before their communications were published.

"The curiously sparse occurrence of the bacilli in lupus suggests a ready explanation of some of the negative results of other histologists, and likewise forbids the hope of deriving material help in diagnosis from the use of the microscope. So far as I am aware, bacilli have not been demonstrated in connection with lupus erythematosus.

"3. *Experimental.*—Koch made inoculations from all his seven cases

into the anterior chamber of the
eyes of rabbits. In every case this
was followed by tuberculosis of the
iris, and in those animals which
lived long enough, by general tuberculosis. Numerous tubercle-bacilli were found in these inoculation-
tubercles. From one specimen
(excised from the cheek of a boy
ten years old) he obtained pure
cultures, which were several times
utilized for successful inoculations
on animals.

"Again, Pagenstecher made
three inoculations from conjunctival
lupus into the anterior chamber of
the eyes of rabbits. In two cases he
succeeded ; in one he failed. Micro-
scopical examination of the 2

successful cases by Pfeiffer (Ehrlich's method) exhibited Koch's bacilli, duly recognised as such by Ziegler, Ehrlich, and others. Positive results such as these, coupled with those of Schuller and Hutter, more than counterbalance the negative results announced by Cohnheim, Hansel, and others.

"Two years ago Vidal and Leloir could assert that 'no results have been obtained from the experimental inoculation of animals with lupus.' Gathering together, then, the foregoing evidence, we seem to be guided to the conclusion that lupus is a tuberculosis (scrofulosis) of the skin excited by the tubercle-bacillus. The localization of the bacillus in the skin, and the relatively rare involvement of other organs, constitute the peculiar features of lupus as compared with other forms of tuberculosis. The bacilli of lupus and tubercle are probably the same qualitatively, but there is a quantitative difference which is accentuated by the more unfavorable conditions of nutrition in the colder skin. Complications with tuberculous affections of other organs— *e. g.*, glands, joints, bones, and even with analogous skin affections— *e. g.*, ulcerating scrofuloides, are frequent. Their non-occurrence does not contradict the tuberculous aetiology of lupus.

"Genetically, then, there is only one tuberculosis of the skin, and we may say that while lupus is always tuberculosis of the skin, yet tuberculosis of the skin assumes other forms than that of lupus (Neisser).

'In short, the evidence is strong of the unity of cause in tuberculosis, lupus, and scrofulosis, although we do not yet know the special determining conditions of each case. Ewald even goes so far as to suggest *Morbus Kochii* as a clinical term for this group of three, by way of analogy to Morbus Brightii, but this innovation is scarcely likely to be approved. The subjoined table may be useful for reference :—

TUBERCULOSIS OF THE SKIN.

1. Miliary Tuberculosis.	2. Lupus (Tuberculo-derma).	3. Ulcerating Scrofulo-derma.
Miliary Tubercles and ulcers as part of a general tuberculosis. Caseates. Very rare.	A harmless (quoad system) form of tuberculosis, mostly limited to the skin. Does not caseate.	i. e., ulcerations arising from bursting of a "cold" subcutaneous abscess. Often yields well to treatment.

Symmetrical.	Unsymmetrical.
Lupus erythematosus. L. sebaceus, etc. Very difficult to cure.	Lupus vulgaris. L. exulcerans, etc. Local Malignancy.

Aberrant forms.

"If asked for a definition of lupus, I would say it is 'a very chronic new cell-growth, depending upon infection with the bacillus tuberculosis, always ending by scars, with or without ulceration, and usually developing brownish-red nodules.''

Now, one would naturally say that if the aetiology of lupus be, as Dr. Smith avers, really to be referred to the same bacillus as that of miliary tuberculosis, then it must be simply a local affection, and the disease would be cured by extrenal local treatment. And Dr. Smith is true to this view, for he says, "It will be generally admitted that local treatment is

the more important." But this is
not *my* experience, for I have never
seen a single case of lupus really
cured by local treatment, though
I have sometimes seen the morbid
process stopped by very severe
cautery or excision ; though even
these severe measures commonly
fail completely.

It is very difficult to cure lupus
by internal medications, but it can
be done ; and Dr. Smith himself
quotes Dr. J. Warburton Begbie
as mentioning that many years ago,
when a student in Paris, he saw
numerous cases of ulcerating lupus
in the wards of St. Louis' Hospital,
which were materially benifited,
and some apparently cured, by the

administration of cod-liver oil in very large doses, and that Dr. Todd Thomson was extremely successful in temporarily, and sometimes even permanently, arresting the ravages of lupus,—undoubted improvement following the use of certain remedies, "chiefly iodine, iron and arsenic conjointly, while local applications were sparingly used."

Although Dr. Smith believes lupus to be dependent upon the tuberculosis bacilli, still he says :— " . . . On the whole, in reference to the internal medication of lupus, we cannot maintain that as yet we know of any specific against the lupus (*i. e.*, tuberculosis) virus ; and perhaps the most that can be done in this way is by strengthening the constitution to increase the capacity for resistance of the body against the spread of the germs of the disease."

We see the Prefossor is slightly befogged in his notions as soon as he touches the art of *Curing !*

Tout comme les autres !

Now, either lupus is, or is not, due to the same bacillus as tuberculosis ; and if so, what relation does the lupus-bacillus bear to the lupus-virus ? or are we to consider bacillus and virus the same thing ?

If lupus is ever to be cured it must be cured by *internal* medication in some *direct* way by a medicament, or by medicaments, standing in *some* relationship to the *whole* lupus process ; to pretend to cure it by killing the bacilli is like the grand old way of catching sparrows by putting salt on their tails.

Case of Generalized Favus.

If there be any one disease of the skin more than another to which one might accord the quality of being *local* and *external*, it is certainly *Favus* ; and yet I read in the *London Medical Record* under the heading of "Case of Generalized Favus" (August 15, 1885), that—

"Professor Kaposi (*Wein. Medizin. Presse*, Oct. 26, 1884) exhibited at the Medical Society of Vienna a remarkable case of favus in which the disease was present on many parts of the skin.

"The patient having died of phlegmonous inflammation of the popliteal space, the autopsy was made by Professor Kundrat, who found that there was *favus of the stomach*. In the neighbourhood of the pylorus there was a patch of infiltration about the size of a 2-franc piece, covered with necrosed tissue 2 millimetres thick. In the exudation, spores and mycelium were found analogous to those present on the skin. It was not found in the intestine. The fungus appears to have provoked the disease of the stomach. The man had been a drunkard, and it is probable that the acidity of the gastric juice was sufficiently diminished to admit of the fungus developing,—an explanation which, however, Professor Bamberger refused to admit."

In this case it would have been eminently instructive if Professor Kaposi (who treats almost every skin disease as a *local* affection) had given the treatment of the defunct Favus-bearer. That the treatment *was* local is almost certain. Moreover, one very naturally asks, of *what nature* was the inflammation of the contents of the popliteal space?

Tumours and the Skin.

An eminently instructive case came under my observation on

August 13, 1885. A lady, just over 50 years of age, came to consult me with regard to a tumour in her right breast, I having successfully treated a lady friend of hers for a similar affection. But it is not about this tumour, as such, that I wish to speak, —it is the antecedent constitutional condition of the patient that bears on my present thesis, viz., the systemic nature of skin diseases. Well, this lady had suffered from red angry pimples on her face, chin, chest, and back all her menstrual life, with coincident neuralgia of right ovary. She had in vain used washes, ointments, and baths for the skin ; only temporary ease and amelioration resulted. But about a year before the date of his visit, she fell with her right breast against a bedstead, and a few months later she noticed a hard lump in her right breast, and her family physician, with a consultant, urged immediate operation, to avoid which she came to me. Just as postscripts are said to contain the real *raison d'etre* of a given epistle, so the parting observation of a patient often throws a strong light on a case. And so here. As she rose from her chair to go, she said. " . . . It is very funny, doctor, but my skin has been so much clearer since the lump came,— in fact, I have very few pimples now; I dare say that has nothing to do with it, but I thought I'd just mention it."

Precisely.

If I have in the foregoing pages succeeded in showing that diseases of the skin are really diseases *of* the system, though *on* the skin, then my task is accomplished. In the near future I hope we may have some *definite* conception of the correspondences that undoubtedly exist between certain regions of the body surface and the internal organs, independently of general organismic interdependence, and then we shall, perhaps, be able to see why certain cutaneous diseases affect certain parts preferentially, and also why, when these diseases are driven in whence they came, by external means, certain internal organs have to bear the brunt of it.

Fletcher's "Etiology."

In his "Elements of General Pathology," p. 99, this great thinker says, in regard to the etiology of skin diseases, "Certain other peculiarities of diet, as the use of cream, cheese, honey, cucumbers, the kernels of fruits, etc., are a frequent exciting cause, according to the idiosyncrasy of the individual, of uticaria, lepra, pityriasis, pomphylix, and other cutaneous eruptions, all which seem to rise in these cases from sympathy with the stomach ; and it is thus that psoriasis, acne, etc., result from cold drinks taken when the stomach is hot."

So that, at least in such cases
as Fletcher cites, if the treatment
is to be local, in what condition is
the stomach left ? and which is the
locus morbi, the stomach or the skin?

I am myself very much dis-
posed to regard what Fletcher calls
"the idiosyncrasy of the individual"
as a *pathic* idiosyncrasy such as, for
example, exists in those persons
who are subject to hay fever.

Acne from Cold Drinks.

In this little volume, I am, before all things, seeking to show that
Diseases of the Skin have, for the
most part, their origin, not in the
skin itself, but are essentially cutaneous manifestations of some

more or less remote organic or organismic wrongs.

Thus Fletcher mentions *Acne from Cold Drinks*, and anent this I wish here to quote an interesting and instructive experience of my own of the curative effects of the *Common Daisy* in complaints that are due to *wet cold—e. g.,* acne of the face.

As I consider the observation of wider practical importance, I will give the source of my own knowledge.

Bellis Perennis against the Ill-Effects of Wet Cold in the Overheated.

I refer to "D. Johann Schroeder's Pharmacopoeia Universalis"

(with Hoffmann's Remarks), Nurn-
berg, 1748. The Daisy is here
commended in Haemorrhage, Dysentery, as a "*herrliches Wund kraut*,"
internally and externally,—*i. e.*, as
a vulnerary,—for the effects of
falls, blows, bruises and the like,
pains in the joints, rheumatism (and
hence called "*Gicht kraut*"), in nocturnal cramps, *angina pectoris*, fevers
and inflammations ; for lameness ;
and he says that German mothers
were in the habit of using it for
their children as an aperient.

An ordinary commendation of
Arnica reads almost in the same
terms, but what I would specially
call attention to is this—"This
herb is useful to such as have

partaken of a too cold draught of
something, for it possesses a peculiar quality, as shown by experience,
of being useful in all those terrible
and dangerous accidents that arise
from having drunk something very
cold when the body is in a heated
condition." This important point
I have verified, as will be seen
later on.

Further, it would appear that
Mindererus, in his *Kriegs-Artzeney*,
cannot sufficiently praise the Daisy
in such cases, for he declares that
an account of this action of the
herb *should be written up over all
gates and doors for the benefit of the
poor harvesters who in the hot har-
vest season get ill from pertaking of*

cold drink ; its effect in such cases he affirms is remarkable, and so prompt that amelioration sets in at once.

Christoph Schorer, in his *Medicina peregrinantium,* gives similar testimony, and says that he cured two men of dangerous coughs, with emaciation, that were due to their having drunk something cold when they were heated. And Schroeder affirms that it will cure dropsy due to drinking too much in "dog days,"—*i. e.,* hot weather.

We know from experince the immense value of certain generalizations in the treatment of disease, as, for instance, *Arnica* for falls and bruises ; *Hypericum* for wounded nerve tissue ; *Dulcamara* for the ill effects of damp, and so on.

Now we may add this other, that *Bellis perennis* is a curative of complaints due to drinking cold drinks when the body is heated,— *i. e.*, Effect of sudden chill from wet cold when one is hot.

Of the use of *Bellis* for the ill effects of cold water suddenly brought into contact with a heated body, I offer the following instructive Case. I will call it

Habitual Periodical Facial Dermatitis.

Miss P., aet. 30, came under my observation on September 24th,

1879, and gave the following history :—Ever since she was 12 years old she had been subject to an eruption of great bumps in the face about every three weeks, sometimes less, sometimes more ; at one time barely to be seen, at another looking like Phlegmonous Erysipelas. This eruption coincided with the commencement of the menstruation. Going back to its origin, I elicited the following curious fact :—

Just before her twelfth year, she was one day out in the fields in sultry weather at hay-making, and while thus greatly heated she fell head foremost into a brook ; and some days thereafter she broke out

all over head and face with an
eruption "just like small-pox."
Her whole face and ears were
covered, and discharged so much
that her mother had to tie a hand-
kerchief round her neck to prevent
its dropping on her clothes. She
was indoors eight weeks with it.
"Since then," shs exclaims, "I
have had any amount of medicines
and greases, and all sorts of things,
but they never did me one bit of
good!" She had often a terrible
sinking at the stomach, as if she
had a large hole wanting filling
up, together with a pressive headache at the top. Bowels regular,
menses very painful—a hot, bad
pain across the hypogastrium at
the beginning.

The *present state* of the face is just this :—The right cheek and right side of the face generally are occupied by a red, tuberous eruption, some of the angry protuberances being as large as big peas, and some only papules, and every size between. Nosologically : *Periodical Dermatitis.*

Now, as to the remedy. I was greatly struck with the history of the case, and I reasoned thus: It arose primarily from the effect of cold water applied to the heated surface of the body (or rather conversely), and that must surely be very like drinking cold water when overheated, and that brought Johannes Schroeder's observation to my mind, viz., that *Bellis* was considered a capital remedy for such as had partaken of cold drink when the body was over-heated. This is, of course, an extension of his application of its use, but the same idea underlies it. How do we know but cold drink taken into a heated body produces internal erysipelas ? If, in the end, this idea be found to bear useful therapeutic fruit, it will doubtless be found in strict conformity with the law of similars. All my observations tend to that conclusion. But considering *Bellis perennis* as analogous in its action to *Arnica* gives a fair reason for its use in this case, as *Arnica* both causes and cures Erysipelas.

Therefore ℞. *Tc. Bellis per.* 3ˣ
ʒiv.

S.—Three drops in water three
times a day.

Oct. 22nd.—Face is quite well;
has not had a speak for the past
fortnight or more. It left gradua-
lly. She is actually; menstrua-
ting (it began yesterday), and
her face is quite free for the first
time at the beginning of the flow
in her whole menstrual life, which
began *eighteen years* ago !! Her
bowels have become *confined*, and
she has now, but only after food,
*a queer shaking, beginning in the
pit of the stomach, and going up to
the throat*, precisely as if she had
been **running fast.**

To take two drops only once a day, and come again in five weeks.

Nov. 24th.—Has continued well of the eruption ; last poorly time not a spot !

She came occasionally for two or three months to report herself, and thus I can affirm that it so far remained permanently cured.

The *Bellis* did *not* affect either the sinking at the stomach or the pressive headache on the top of the head at all ; so, early in december, I gave her *Sulphur 30*, *one drop* at bedtime for twelve days, when these two symptoms also disappeared. It is to be noted that these two symptoms were of much later date than the facial dermatitis.

Of course, my reasoning in the foregoing case might be faulty, but I think it shows that the Daisy is a notable remedy, and this virtue of a common weed lying everywhere at our feet deserves to be made very widely known. People of any experience do not need to be told that the ill effects of drinking cold drinks when the body is heated are very serious at times, and always inconvenient. Of course it is not confined to the drinking, as the idea is *sudden wet chill to heated stomach* or *body surface*. This property of the daisy is the more valuable, as we know of no other remedy in our vast Pharmacopoeia that possesses it ; and, beyond myself, I believe no

one is acquainted with it. Most
of what I here write has been
lying in a drawer of my writing-
desk for years, and this little
clinical tip ought long since
to have been published, for
it may be a good while before
another lover of the fair Daisy
stumble against old Schroeder's
generalization in a humble recep-
tive mood. I regard this peculiar
property of the Daisy as eminently
important, and ask all who may
read this to make it known, so
that it may be available for such
as travellers, tourists, harvesters,
soldiers on the march, when they,
being heated, have had a cold
ducking, or have drunk cold
liquids.

I would recommend it also in the acute and chronic dyspepsia from eating cold ices, as the conditions here are identical, for I have, in such cases, found it an eminent curative agent.

I should like very much to dilate on the remarkable therapeutic virtues of the Daisy, but this is not the place. This much is, however, apposite, for the Facial Dermatitis was one that would certainly be classed as a Disease of the Skin, and internal treatment alone cured it.—Q. E. D.

Quite lately I have information of the cure by *Bellis perennis* of a severe case of Facial Acne, produced originally by patient's rushing about in the cold air while her face was in a very heated condition.

PART II.

OBJECTIONS to the first edition of this little treatise were raised largely because of its essentially theoretical character ; well, that is really a compliment to the writer, whose object was to point out how entirely wrong are the commonly accepted views as to the nature and cure of cutaneous affections, and not to show that X cures Y. In some cases of disease it may, perhaps, not very much signify what views of aetiology and pathology the treating physician may have ; but I submit it makes all the difference

in the world when we are dealing
with skin diseases. If the position
which I take up be the true one,
skin doctors are working great
evil in the world, and sadly need
enlightening ; while, on the other
hand, if they are right, and their
almost universally accepted views
and practice are sound and in
accordance with the facts of disease,
then I must be in the worng, and
wrong should every-where be
crushed like a nut under a steam-
hammer. Dermatologists ! I ask
no mercy, as I give no quarter.

Sine Ira et Studio.

We all subscribe to this saying,
sine ira et studio, but in the search
after light and real facts we are all

apt to become merely advocates of
our own pet notions. Said a gentleman to me one day, "Doctor, I
have read your book ; you ought
to have been an advocate ; I do not
know about your *facts* !" With
that he ran off laughing, and was
clearly of opinion that he left me at
full length in the dust. Well,
thought I, I will consider afresh the
whole question of Diseases of the
Skin from the standpoint of the
organism as an entirety, and as my
little book on the subject, published
in 1886, is out of print, and my publishers are asking for a new edition,
I will give just a few of the results
of my reconsideration in this second
edition. Here they are. By the
way, the clinical material made use

of in the first edition came down to the commencement of the year 1885, so far as my own case-takings in my own practice were concerned, and at this point I will resume my task.

Case of Ichthyosis.

A lady of 73 years of age came to consult me in the month of March 1885 for loss of vision due to double cataract. In dealing with cataract I always go at once to a consideration of the skin, and here the find was instructive ; her skin was very thick, dry, hot, and scaly, notably on the extensor surfaces, with long cracks here and there. In her movements patient is exceedingly slow, spending as much as two hours at her very simple morning toilet. Though her skin had never been other than dry and scaly, it is getting much worse of late years. Her lenses were opaque and of a milky colour, and the epidermic scales light-coloured, though not particularly pearl-like,—just a case of chronic diffuse hypertrophic keratosis.

This lady has continued under my observation up to the present time, and so would now be in her 79th or 80th year. She was nearly blind when she came to me, being just able to find a large object; thus with a little groping and feeling with her knees she could find a chair to sit upon. There were temporary improvements in vision here and there, and the lady has still a very small amount of vision. But on the other hand, there has been a very distinct imrovement in her skin, which is neither so thick nor so scaly, nor so much cracked. And considering the age of the patient and the very long duration of the affection, I think the improvement in her skin very noteworthy indeed, and her various ailings have been from time to time much relieved as well. During the five and a half years she had from me many remedies,— *Calcarea fluorica 6, Psoricum 30, Natrum muriaticum 30, Psor. c., Thuja 30, Lactuca vir. 3,*

Galium aparine **1ˣ**, *Platanus occidentalis* **1ˣ**, *Graphites* **30**, *Ichthyol* **30**, *Baryta mur.* **3ˣ**, and here—August, 1887— there was very distinct amelioration both in the skin and lenses. *Calcarea hypophosphorosa* **3ˣ**, *Aconitum* **3ˣ**, *Aurum muriaticum natronatum* **3ˣ**. *Pulsatilla*, *Bryonia*, *Borax*, *Betula alba* θ, *Juglans cinerea*.

The remedies that were of very distinct advantage were *Barium* and *Platanus*. Under *Barium* for several months patient increased in vigour and well-being, and under the *Platanus* for several months also her skin admittedly underwent considerable improvement.

The *Betula alba* patient credited with rendering the skin much more comfortable, but complained that it affected the upper part of the body only.

A friend of this aged lady spoke slightingly of the treatment of this case, inferring that as the case was not cured, the whole thing was a fiasco. But I pointed out that what results from the treatment is strong evidence of beneficial drug-action in a very inveterate case at an advanced age ; that the lady's discomforts have been greatly alleviated ; that at 78 her skin is actually *much better* than it was at 73 ; while at 73 it was getting worse and worse, her skin at 78 is not getting worse, but better.

The fact that the lady's span of life is dwindling has nothing to do with the clinical evidence of curative results from drug-action, or rather the greater the age of the patient the more remarkable the evidence. We must remember that what we call life is to each individual of us a varying quantity, according to our respective ages, and at 78 life to this lady is *what remains to come after 78 !* It may not be much, but it is *life to her :* in other words, alleviating an old patient is, medically speaking, not diminished because the patient benefited may not have long to live by reason of advanced age, —

"At six I well remember when
All folks seemed old at ten."

Severe Case of Eczema of Sixteen Years' Standing—Elephantiasis Labiorum Vulvæ—Life-long Constipation.

A strong, well-preserved lady, 70 years of age, came under my observation on October 9th, 1890, telling me she had very severe eczema for the last sixteen years, and now for some time past has what has been called dry ecxema of the vulvar lips, and there is also a patch of "dry eczema" over her right eye. Both the vulvar lips of the right side were hugely enlarged, and appeared as a big flap of elephantine nature, scaly, shiny, deeply pigmented, reddish in spots, dry and itchy. Patient, though English and long resident in England, is, nevertheless, of West India birth, having left her birthplace and came to this country at the age of 6 years, —*i. e.*, sixty-four years ago. I mention this point because I do not remember ever seeing a case like this before, and hence presume it cannot be common in London, or generally in this country. The irritation was very bad ; worse after sitting or walking much, and also at night, when it keeps her awake ; it is much worse in the cold weather, diminishing much in the warm weather of summer. Patient enjoyed good health, and has never had anything beyond measles, scarlatina, and pertussis. She complains of being chilly. Nothing seemed to account for so severe an affection in an otherwise strong, healthy lady. There had been in all three vaccinations, the third one having been unsuccessful, and was in 1871. The eczema had first obtruded itself upon patient's attention sixteen years ago,—*i. e.*, subsequent to this third unsuccessful vaccination.

Thuja 30.

October 30, 1890.—The little patch of eruption over the eye is well, the labial swelling is less, the mass softer, and patient exclaimed, "I feel quite different."

℞. *Sabina* 30.

November 20.—Not any further improvement.

℞. *Vaccininum* 30.

December 18.—The bowels have acted twice every day, and she had been costive all her life ; has been always in the habit of going six or seven days without any motion, and then art and physic had to do it. "Dr. Bell (homoeopath) theated my constipation for long, and finally gave it up as a constitutional peculiarity."

℞. *Maland. CC.*

January 8, 1891.—Patient cried out to me on this day :—"English, French, German, allopathic and homoeopathic,— all have tried at my costiveness in vain, and now the bowels act *so* well." The elephantine skin of labia steadily improving.

February. 5—skin healing well ; bowels not quite so comfortable.

℞. *Vaccininum 30.*

Feb. 26.—Skin affection improving ; bowels act comfortably. "I have never felt so well in my life."

℞. *Nux* 30, under which the bowels went back.

March 19.—*Vaccin.*, *30.*

May 21.—Well ; bowels act quite regularly and comfortably ; and though patient feels not quite comfortable at the vulva, objectively the skin is quite normal.

At the end of November the skin continued quite normal, and hence we may conclude that the cure is a perfect one.

Nine months Later.—The cure holds good. And this radical cure of an old-standing ailment in a lady of 70 years of age,—the remedies used being all given internally, and not only so, but in dynamic doses (and frequently),—this cure, I say, is noteworthy, and tells well for my thesis that skin diseases are of constitutional nature, and must be so regarded and treated. *Natura* [*organismus*] *sanat, madicus curat.*

Case of Acne And Swelled Neck.

On February 10, 1891, an unmarried lady, well on towards 30, came to consult me for roughness of the skin of the face, and acne. She did not mind her cough, it was not so very bad, nor did she make much ado about the rather profuse expectoration of phlegm. She did

not even complain of her enlarged
tonsils or leucorrhoea, and as for
her chilblains, they only came in
very cold weather. Said she, "It
is my rough skin and this horrid
neck." The "horrid neck" was
made up of a one-sided enlargement of the neck, consisting of a
very much hypertrophied submaxillary gland and tonsil of the
same side, with some puffiness of
the surrounding areolar tissue, so
that the side of the neck appeared
"horrid,"—*i. e.*, shapeless, and
neck and face ran into one another,
the jaw-bone line being lost. *Thuja
30* for a month distinctly lessened
the size of the glands (submaxillary and tonsil), but cough and
phlegm were not touched.

Bacillinum C. was followed by much improvement, the unshapeliness having changed : the jaw had become well defined, and thus neck and face no longer ran into one another, while the left submaxillary gland stood out by itself. The tonsils had gone down, but the quantity of phlegm, though less, was still considerable. I then went up to *Bac.* 1000. "Those powders did a wonderful thing for my skin : it went quite clear"

July 21, 1891.—Patient is quite well ; skin clear ; tonsils normal ; left submaxillary enlargement gone ; neck restored to its pristine shapeliness ; and not long after this she was engaged to be married, and in the early autumn the marriage came off.

My reading of the whole case was to the effect that I was dealing with vaccinosis and scrofulosis bordering on tuberculosis. May I put pertinent question to any dermatologist or surgeon in this wide world of ours : What would you have done in this case ?

August 1892.—Patient continues quite well, as I learn from her mother, lady X.

Ulcerative Eruption of Vulva.

A lady of 50 years of age, for many years married, but childless, came under my care for troubles connected with the climaxis, not

10

the least of which was vaginal and vulvar irritation, as well as a very extensive ulcerative erpution all over the labial and vulvar region extending at times as far as an inch and a half on to the circumvulvar region, but when it came into the common intigument it took more the form of eczema, with a few pustules here and there. The flat ulcers in the labia and nymphae had plagued her years ago, and been cured (silenced) by cauterization. ℞ *Tc. Platin. Mur.* 3ˣ, three drops in water twice a day.

In a month the eruption had materially diminished, having lost its pustular and purulent character, and the vaginal discharge had entirely ceased.

Here (*May* **27**, 1887) *Lachesis* was ordered, and with advantage.

July. 7, 1887.—The ;thing has returned.

℞ *Tc. Aurum mur. nat.* **3ˣ**, four drops in a tablespoonfull of water night and morning.

This completely cured the eruption with its concomitants, the remedy having to be once subsequently repeated: in all, the *Auric salt* was taken during, about thirteen or fourteen weeks. There has been no return, and the lady continues in excellent health and condition. I used no local application whatever. And here I may state, once for all, that I hardly ever order local applications of any sort in cutaneous

affections. If in any of my cases
herein recited any local applications are used, the fact will be stated; but I believe in no case herein
communicated was any local application whatever used, so far as I am
aware. Not only so, but I commonly
specially warn my patients against
all ointments and lotions whatever,
as I find that Goulard's lotion, Zinc
ointment, Citrine ointment, Golden
ointment, and the like, may be
found in very many households, and
it is very difficult to prevent their
being used.

The use of remedies applied as
ointments or lotions is absolutely
bad; and when I read of the homoeopathic treatment of skin diseases whereby ointments and lotions

play a part, my respect for the quality of such treatment is small indeed. It is wonderful how people will cuddle and fondle the ointment pot; and "Regular Medicine" would be indeed badly off without its grease pot and clyster. I often think the use by the homoeopaths of their *Calendula cerate* or ointment comes dangerously near the thin end of the wedge of the vulgarly-conceived putty-and-paint treatment of the medicines of the schools.

It is almost incredible, but the discovery of a new fat for an unguental excipient is an event of the first ·magnitude in the dermatological world, the vault of whose heaven is still ringing with the

echoes of the wonders of veseline
and lanoline. And what does it all
amount to ?

A pat of pig's lard.

Case of Pityriasis Rubra.

Although the Vienna School
classifies this rather rare affection
with eczema, I cannot see myself
whereon the classification is based;
but I have only had to treat two
typical cases of it, both being of
the cutaneous covering of the chest,
and two or three cases of symptoms of the rim of the hairy scalp,
which were distinctly of the same
nature. The patient here referred
to came to me on December 22,

1885. A powerful peer of this realm
and a great Nimrod, with flesh as
hard as nails, he came to be treated
for a maddening neuralgia he had
picked up on the banks of the Nile;
remedies having cured his neuralgia he showed me his chest, which
was the seat of a big patch of red
pityriasis that he had had for a
number of years,—the precise number I do not know. I saw him, off
and on, for nearly five years, and
gave him a not inconsiderable portion of our Pharmacopoeia (and
our Pharmacopoeia is not small
—*see* Allen's "Encyclopaedia of
Pure Materia Medica !"), but the
pityriasis rubra remained . . . .
Pityriasis rubra. I should say the
big patch was composed of a series

of smaller patches, all more or less circular or segments of circles.

One day I was reading in an old German Book that some sailors—British, I think—many years ago, in some of the Pacific islands, ate of a fish called erythrinus, and came out with a peculiar red rash that became chronic, and which the doctors took for a form of syphilis.

Dr. Alfred Heath, F. L. S., with his wonted devotion and disinterestedness, procured this erythrinus for me, and prepared it homoeopathically, and I, on March 23, 1889, ordered as follows : ℞ *Tc. Erythrinus* 1 ℥j., five drops in water night and morning. I did not see the patient after for about two and a half years—viz., September 1, 1891. When I inquired of him about the "red patch of his chest," "Oh," said he, "you cured that long ago with that big bottle of stuff you sent me, " *i. e.*,— the ounce bottle of *Erythrinus 1*.

The second case of pityriasis which I treated with this *Erythrinus* is greatly improved, but by no means cured. The father of the gentleman who was cured by *Erythrinus* had had syphilis, as I ascertained from an indirect but very reliable source.

The father of the second case died of what seems to have been aneurism of or near the heart. It may therefore be worth while to ascertain whether pityriasis rubra be not a syphilitic manifestation in the second generation. That it is not eczema I am very sure. It is worthy of note that the second patient to whom I here refer,—who is not cured, and is still under my treatment,—came to me originally for heart disease characterized by distress in the heart region, palpitation, irregular heart-beat, and much distress on walking, particularly up hill.

For this cardiac affection (which the regimental surgeon said would be fatal) I prescribed *Aurum muriaticum* 3ˣ, at one time three drops, and at another time two drops, and finally five drops, in a

table spoonful of water three times
a day. This cured the heart rather
slowly, but the patch of pityriasis
became twice as large. This vicarious
phenomenon between heart and
the skin of the thorax I have
observed over and over again. So
that when an individual has an
eruption on his chest, he is not wise
to let any skin specialist treat it
from the narrow standpoint of the
specialist, lest heart disease supervene. See here anent my remarks
upon the "Sternal Patch." By the
way the "Sternal Patch" is in the
lowest third of the sternum, rather
to the right ; this thoracic pityriasis
patch is rather to the left, and just
over the arch of the aorta. The
"Sternal Patch" is not a brown,

so-called, liver mark, but an eruption ; the importance of this eruption lies, I think, not so much in the kind of eruption as in the fact that when it vanishes from the surface, without being really cured from within, symptoms of heart disease, more or less grave, at once supervene. The more one really studies skin diseases the more one is struck with their *habitats*, which are often constant and characteristic. What are the internal pathological conditions corresponding hereto ? Without doubt such exist, and have also a definite significance.

Case of Violent and Severe Attacks of Arthritic Urticaria.

A lady of position, nearing 70 years of age, of very abstemious habits and a strict dietarian, had been for years subject to violent and severe attacks of gouty nettle-rash, taking her suddenly, now in one part, now in another, and compelling her to hasten to her own apartments to apply hot wraps to allay the furious itching. She had been under most of the better-known homoeopathic physicians in England one time and another, and had obtained a little temporary relief sometimes, but not much, so that she had given up all hope for long, and only consented to try again at the earnest solicitation of a friend. When she took my prescription into her hand, she exclaimed, "Oh! that's your tincture of nettles : that's no good. I have tried that under Dr.——,and my dear old friend the late Dr. Hilbers also gave it to me." She persisted in it that *Urtica* would do her no good, but I persuaded her to take it *(Urtica urens* θ), five drops in a wine-glassful of warm water three times a day ; and much to her surprise, it did her so much good that she continued to take it for some months, and then discontinued its use, considering herself cured.

In connection with this case it is worth remembering that *Urtica* had in old times quite a reputation for gout and sand, and I have repeatedly noticed that patients, while taking *Urtica ur.* θ in the manner just described, have passed large quantities of sand, and in

several instances such patients
have been alarmed, never having
passed any before in their lives.

Urtica urens is a very notable
splenic, and with its aid I have
often cured ague. And for the
common manifestations of pure
gout, it is my sheet-anchor for years
past. I could fill a little book with
cases in proof of this statement.

Dyspepsia—Vomiting—Neuralgia
Neurasthenia—Acute Eczema.

A married lady, childless, 55
years of age, came to me on July
12, 1887, quite broken down in
health ; it was thought the final
break-up of the constitution was at
hand. The most prominent and

most distressing symptom was
perhaps her attacks of faintness
and her inveterate and severe dyspepsia, though she felt her nerve
symptoms very much. She was
afraid of being alone, going about
in fear and trembling. Nervous
heart-beat ; spleen very much enlarged (affirmed that she had had
ague every spring until she was
nearly thirty years of age) ; a good
deal of neuralgia in the left side of
head and face. She is intolerant of
Cold, and revels in this July heat.
This lady is an amateur artist, and
paints a good deal these many years,
and wonders if her frequent attacks
of vomiting have any connection
there with. She formerly had vari-
ola and measles, and has also

suffered from urticaria. But the fact that she had been twice vaccinated seemed to me the most proximate and least questionable therapeutic indication. Hence I started off with *Thuja 30*.

August 11.—Was quite well till two days ago! No vomiting; slight neuralgia only; no fainting attacks; tongue now thickly coated.

The next most obvious point to attack was the greatly enlarged spleen and the chilliness.

℞. *Caenothus Americanus* 1. Six drops in water night and morning.

December 1.—My patient came this day and bitterly complained that the *Ceanothus* had done no good at all, and had, moreover, brought back all the old symptoms, which the *Thuja* powder had so much benefitted. The neuralgia is bad again, and patient very earnestly requests that she have the old powders again.

So *Thuja 30* was again prescribed in very infrequent doses.

January 17, 1888.—Has a bad attack now on these eight days, and there is a little eruption on the tips of her toes and fingers; no vomiting.

℞ *Ignatia amara 1.*

February 19.—Much better; in fact, feels wonderfully well, *but she has "broken out all over with an eruption of water and matter."* And

she now has ceased to be cold, and
is, on the contrary *hot*.

℞. *Tc. Juglans regia* θ. Five
drops in water night and morning.

March 27.—The skin has improved a good deal; as the eruption
dies away the locus turns brown;
the eruption is now worse on the
hairy scalp; she feels sick and
dizzy. Never had any eruption
other than urticaria till after she
took the *Thuja* from me. Much
better in all general respects.

℞. *Rep.*

May 8.—Been sick again, three
times; many brown marks where
the eruption was, otherwise she is
well and the skin is quite healthy.

The spleen, however, continues hypertrophied.

℞. *Urtica urens* θ. Five drops in water night and morning.

October 6.—Bowels costive; feels tired and bilious, and complains very much of feeling shivery and cold *Natrum muriaticum* 6 trituration cured these symptoms, and patient was discharged cured.

July 1893.—The cure holds good.

Case of Strumous Eczema in a Baby, cured by *Bacillinum* CC.

One meets not infrequently with bad cases of eczema in babies that are apt to end in marasmus and death : the eruption in such cases is almost all over the body, wetting, more particularly in certain more or less circumscribed patches, and driving the poor little patients almost mad with irritation, particularly at night. I had such a case this last summer in a baby of only a few months of age, and who was partly on the cursed bottle. Did I say cursed bottle ? I will withdraw the wicked word and ask my readers to allow me to substitute for it——, well, I mean the strongest word of condemnation known in our language. In this particular case the mother did her best, so the use of the bottle could not be avoided, and its use was only partail, the mother giving all she had.

Well, I had treated the eczema for some weeks with no benefit, when one afternoon I was suddenly summoned into the country to see this poor bairnie, and a sorry sight it was.

Mother and nurse were at their wit's end to know how to keep the wet patches from sticking to the clothes, fat-besmeared rags only sufficing for a very short time. Hardly any sleep at night from the furious irritation. I then remembered that I once cured an elder baby-brother of this little patient of eczema of the scalp with *Bacillinum*, originally suggested by the ancient scars in their father's neck, now well hidden behind his long beard   therefore ordered for my wee patient *Bacill. CC.* in infrequent doses.

In one week the report ran : ". . . Baby is much better, and now sleeps and feeds beautifully."

I need only add that the remedy quite cured the case, and the little lassie got quite well, and so remains.

Such cases are very apt to end fatally, whereof I have been in times past more than once the sorrowful witness ; but then I knew nothing of *Bacillinum* in high potency, or, indeed, in any potency.

The patient in question had not at that period been vaccinated.

Inveterate Eczema.

An American gentleman, 63 years of age, came under my

observation on May 14, 1887, for a very severe eruption on the skin — inveterate eczema—of many years' duration. Latterly it has been getting much worse and more extensive, and extends now to the penis, prepuce, and eyelids and conjunctivae. There was a specific air about it, but this was strictly denied, a gonorrhoea only being admittedly historic.

I began with *Platanus occidentalis* θ, but in eight days from its commencement patient returned to me, bitterly complaining that there was no improvement.

May 21.—Six grains of *Aurum metallicum* three times a day. This did him some good certainly, but not very much. Then followed *Mercurius solubilis Hahn.* in a low trituration, and it was soon clear that we had hold of the right remedy, but it would not quite finish the cure, though it came very near doing so. A month of *Kali chlor,* 3ˣ, and patient considered himself cured, except the redness of the eyes. This ophthalmia was cured by *Jequirity* 3ˣ, six drops in water night and morning.

I saw this gentleman a year and a half later, when he declared himself quite well in health and free from eczema.

Case of Gouty Eczema.

In the autumn of 1891 a gentleman of about 60 years of age consulted me in regard to a very severe form of eczema occupying the genital, perineal, anal, and crural regions : the surface was red, raw, shiny, scaly in part, and in part moist. The thing caused him very great distress. The first two prescriptions did him no real good, so on November 27th, 1891, I prescribed the hippurate of sodium in the fifth centesimal dilution in ten-drop doses, administered every night and morning, I sending him enough to last a month.

I saw no more of him till the spring of 1892, and then I inquired of the skin trouble. "Oh ! that tincture cured me completely." To be quite sure it was so, I carefully examined the parts, and I did the same again four months later, when he called to ask me to suggest a place where he might with advantage spend his holiday. I found no trace of eczema on either occasion, and patient continues in good health. I have seen and treated a good many cases of eczema, and am just beginning to recognise its rather numerous varieties from the aetio-pathological standpoint, and I shall yet have more to say on the subject : here let the simple narrative of the case cured by the hippurate of sodium suffice.

Lichen Urticarus.

A sixteen-months' old baby was brought to me by its mother on November 27, 1886, to be treated for wheals on its body that became much worse in the warmth of the bed : the distress of the child was great ; it got hardly any proper sleep.

R. *Syph CC.*

January 13, 1887.—These little powders quite cured baby in less than a fortnight."

August 30, 1887.—"Baby's skin continues quite well."

Cases of wheals in the skin of young children are very common, and the irritation they cause as the sufferers get warm in bed is often almost maddening. I have known such patients toss and roll about almost every night, and not infrequently roll out of bed in their sleep, as if they were making desperate efforts to escape from their tormentors.

Chloral hydrate and *Urtica urens*, and also *Persicaria urens* are very useful in such cases, and so is also *Bacillinum*. But where the nocturnally appearing wheals are, as it were, echoes from the paternal past, nothing equals the remedy here named as curative. The thing is cured root and branch, recurring occasionally when a new tooth sprouts, when the dose has to be repeated once, or perhaps twice, till the cure is definitely completed.

Where the primary causation is from the effects of vaccination, *Thuja, Sabina, Cupressus, Vaccininum,* or *Malandrinum* may be used, *Thuja* generally sufficing; and I have required *Acidum nitricum* in some cases.

Crop of Soft Warts Round the Anus.

A middle-aged married gentleman came under my observation in the summer of 1892 complaining of severe indigestion of long standing : a good deal of epigastric distress and pain characterized his dyspeptic state. Incidentally he complained of a most uncomfortable state of his anal region, and on examining this part to ascertain the cause thereof I found a number of small warts arranged almost in a ring round the orifice. A gonorrhoea

of many years ago, as also several
vaccinations, sufficed to constitute
the diagonosis of Hahnemannic sy-
cosis, and, indeed, *Thuja occid*, in
the 30th centesimal potency, and of
infrequent administration, quite
cured the dyspepsia, and also the
anus. I carefully examined the anal
region, and found that the ring of
small soft warts had quite disappeared. "I feel all right there now."

Nasal Erythema.

A lady, 53 years of age, came
under my professional care in the
summer of 1890, with erythema of
the nose, or, as we might call it,
dermatic rhinitis. The nose was
all red and swelled up, the inflammatory action not in any way ex-

tending to the cheeks, but involving the right eye a good deal. In fact, patient, is of opinion that the right-sided conjunctivitis was the starting point of the nasal erythema, and she tells me that she is subject to this ocular inflammation, off and on, for many years.

Anamnetically there is not much to note, except that the lady had been vaccinated seven or eight times, but it had only taken three times.

Under *Thuja* 30 the erythema was half gone in three weeks, and patient had visibly improved in condition. After two months of the *Thuja* the eye was quite well, the erythema still only half well

Finding that the nose scabbed inside, I put patient on *Kali bichromi-
cum* 5, five drops in water night
and morning for a month, and then
patient was discharged cured. (See
the pathogenesis of *Kali bi.*)

Life-long Eruption on Scalp.

A single gentleman, 35 years of
age, came to consult me at the end
of August 1887 for a coppery
eruption of his scalp that he had
had as long as he could remember.
Besides this eruption he complained
much of chronic insomnia and failing memory. I first gave him the
strong tincture of *Fagus cup.*, five
drops in water night and morning,

but after a month—viz., on September 30—he complained that he was no better in any respect,—sleepless, forgetful, restless; the eruption bad; his breath very foul ; liver slightly enlarged ; spleen large and very hard.

Syp. CC.

Novemeber 11.—"I have slept famously ;" and both he and I were of opinion that his hair had gone darker. The eruption distinctly better.

℞ *Spiritus glandium quercus* θ, five drops in water night and morning.

December 12.—Eruption nearly gone; the spleen pains a little now ; insomnia quite a thing of the past.

℞. *Tc. Carduus Marioe.*

He reported himself quite well of
his coppery eruption on January 13,
1888, and two years later it still
continued well, and since then I
have no further tidings of him.

Chronic Crops of Boils and Acne.

A young city man, 21 years of
age, just entering a very important
city firm, came under my observation
on March 21st, 1888, complaining
that for the past six years he had
been suffering from crops of boils.
They are worse on his nape and face;
at this moment there is one on the
nape, and also one on his nose.
There are also mattery spots—acne
--all over his shoulders. Patient is
very rich and rather good-looking,

8

and it is therefore not astonishing
that he had been under the professional care of the leading physicians
and surgeons and skin specialists
of London, to the number of ten.
Finding quite a goodly collection of vaccinial scars on both
arms, I inquired what number
of times he had been vaccinated.
Answer : Four times. Urine has
a specific gravity of 1020, and the
glands of his neck are visibly
swelled. I had him about ten
weeks under *Thuja occidentalis 30*,
very infrequently administered, and
the boils and acne pustules all waned
and went and came no more, much
to patient's amazement, and, indeed,
to my own, for I had not expected
such a prompt and perfect cure. I

subsequently often saw him with
his younger brother, and so know
that the cure was definite. The case
wase clearly one of pure and uncom-
plicated vaccinosis without the dash
of consumptiveness that so often
lurks behind severe acne.

There is also a kind of acne that
is distinctly of arthritic nature, and
this yields well to *Urea 6* ; in this
variety pustulation is much less pronounced than in vaccinial acne or
phthisic acne. Broadly put, vaccinial acne yields to *Thuja occidentalis, Sabina* and *Cupressus*, also to
Silicea and *Maland* ; acne from
masturbation, to *Bellis perennis* ;
phthisic acne, to *Bacillinum* ; when
the acne is very pronouncedly pustular and scarring, to *Vaccinin*. and

Variolinum; and arthritic acne calls for hippuric acid, hippurate of sodium, and *Urea*. The study of the varieties of acne is highly interesting and instructive, as almost all the great constitutional ancestral diseases show themselves in young persons in the form of acne. Not infrequently cases of acne are of mixed pathological qualities, and these need *all* their pathologic *simillima*. Remedies only morphologically homoeopathic to the acneform only palliate ; to really and radically cure they must be *pathologically* similar. What a vast vista !

Ringworm (Herpes s. Tinea Tonsurans)

This is a very interesting complaint, and particularly so from the biological standpoint ; but as I have written a little monograph on the subject, I must refer my readers to it for the fuller information which it contains. It is entitled "Ringworm : Its Constitutional Nature and Cure" (London, 1892). It is also published in America by Messrs. Boericke & Tafel, and may be obtained at any of their pharmacies.

The order remedies for its cure are *Sepia*, *Sulphur*, and *Tellurium* ; my own special remedy is *Bacillinum* in high potency, which is not merely a morphological simile, but what I conceive to be its pathological *simillimum*.

In treating ringworm cases by *Bacillinum* it must be borne in

mind that the constitutional crasis
is aimed at, and not the parasitic
fungi. This is highly important,
as the following narration will exemplify. Soon after the appearance
of my little work on Ringworm
just referred to, a very eminent
London ringworm specialist, desir-
ous of practically testing my treatment, sent a very delicate, stunted,
strumous girl to me, saying, "Here
is a case after Dr. Burnett's own
heart. Tell him from me that I re-
gret being unable to co-operate with
him, as he is a homoeopath ; but
you go and see what he can do,"

Well, that was, I must confess,
very handsome of him. The
mother brought the girl, and I put
her upon *Baillinum* and gave up

all local treatment altogether. In
the course of about two months the
improvement in the child's general
health was very marked, and the
parents were delighted ; but the
precious fungi on the head haunted
the child's mother so, that although
she was very pleased to admit the
great improvement in the child's
appetite, sleep, temper, and appearance, still she wanted to know from
the said specialist whether the parasitic fungi were decreasing ; and
having taken her to him, it was
found that the head was *much
worse* !—*i. e.*, the number of fungi
was much greater ; and therefore
my plan of treatment was given up
as a dead failure ! It did not occur
to these good people that my stand-

point is the very opposite of theirs :
I deal with the organism, they deal
with the parasites. The organism was admittedly improved, the
number of parasites demonstrably
greater. I claim that the child
was visibly getting better. There
being more parasites, they considered that she was worse, or at
any rate that the ringworm was
worse, although the patient was
better in herself.

Now, I not only do not claim that
the number of parasites and their
spores decrease in the beginning of
my treatment, what I claim is that
eventually they go altogether as
soon as the organism is normally
healthy. Of course, it must be
obvious that there would be fewer

parasites present on the head while it was being scoured twice a day than while the head was let alone entirely. That the number of the parasites and their spores can be kept down by external parasiticidal treatment I do not for one moment dispute ; what I say is, that the parasites themselves are not the disease, but are nearly the tricho-phyton mould living on the surface of a diseased organism; and, further, I incline very strongly to the belief that not only are the fungi harmless to the patient, but probably actually beneficial as organismic scavengers.

Do mushrooms come in a clean new stable, or in a dirty disused one ?

Do toadstools grow on healthy trees, or on decaying ones? Which existed first—the decaying wood or the toadstool? Can you cure a decaying tree by killing the toadstools?

Fungi live on decaying matter, and their function is to use up and get rid of such decay; and I am fully persuaded that the function the trichophyton of ringworm is in harmony with this general principle.

It is inconceivable that you can better the health of a child by cleaning the ringwormy mould off the surface of its body.

It is equally inconceivable that you should be able to keep ringworm alive on a healthy individual, or, if so, then fish can live in the air, and a cow could live the life of a whale.

Alopecia Areata.

This is an affection of the hairy scalp principally, and consists of shiny, bald, circular patches, in appearance not unlike the surface of a billiard ball. I do not think the affection can be considered a common one, though of course a few cases of it constantly pass before us. Authorities differ a good deal about it, particularly as to whether the decalvation be of epiphytic nature or not.

But there is one point in regard to alopecia areata in which all the dermatologists and skin surgeons

agree, and that is their treatment—
viz., active irritants applied to these
bald patches. This treatment is
simple, sometimes painful, me-
chanically childish, and besides being well-nigh universal, is at the
same time quite useless except in
very simple cases. Given a good stiff
case of alopecia araeta, and all the
skin specialists and all the favourite irritants of all the dermatologists
of the wide world cannot cure it.

Hughes names *Phos. acid*, *Fluoric
acid*, and *Arsenic*, and considers
the second-named specific in the
syphilitic form.

Huges also calls attention to
Teste's singular experience with
Aloes.

Goullon (the second) praises *Graphites*, *Baryta carbonica*, *Lycopodium*, *Mercurius*, and *Natrum muriaticum*.

In alopecia areata the only sound plan is to heal the *patient* rather than the alopecia. What the real nature of areata baldness may be is still a moot point. We shall not lose time if we inquire into this point somewhat. Probably few people know more about this subject than Mr. Jonathan Hutchinson, late President of the Royal College of Surgeons. We will therefore consult him on the subject.

On Alopecia Areata and its Relation to Ringworm.

Mr. Jonathan Hutchinson brings forward a series of cases *(Archives of Surgery,* April 1893), altogether 39 in number, of alopecia, and seeks to connect them aetiologically with ringworm. He says he does not think that anyone will read attentively the items of evidence (*i. e.,* these 39 cases) which he brings forward without coming to the same conclusions he has arrived at himself ; and the chief of these conclusions is, that "all well characterised cases of alopecia areata are in direct connection either with ringworm or pityriasis versicolor, and that they have little or nothing to do with the state of the patient's general health."

Our author reckons hereto all cases of loss of hair beginning as smooth bald patches which are abruptly margined, which tend to spread at their edges, and which are attended by the development of others in their vicinity.

'In some cases the patient may lose every hair on the body in the course of a few months, whilst in others the patch may remain single and solitary for a year or more." "Differences in the rate and extent of progress do not seem to me to imply any difference in the essential nature of the disease ; and I much doubt whether there is any class of cases in which the shedding of the hair becomes universal which are not of the nature of alopecia areata."

Alder Smith ("Ringworm : its Diagnosis and Treatment," London, 1885) says alopecia areata "is due to a state of perverted nutrition and not to any vegetable parasite," and refers to a paper read at the International Medical Congress in 1881, on the Cause of Alopecia, by Dr. Liveing, proving its non-parasitic nature.

Alder Smith adds, "It is hardly necessary for me to remark that I fully agree with this view, having never been able to discover any fungus in the club-shaped stumps." So here, on the other hand, alopecia areata is declared to be *non*-parasitic ; and with regard to allowing a child with alopecia into a school, Alder Smith declares "there is no fear of the disease spreading ; and therefore children with alopecia may be allowed to attend school without any risk to others."

The bald patches of alopecia areata commence most commonly at the back of the head, and Mr. Hutchinson thinks this is due to the infection coming from cushions and the backs of chairs.

Bringing ringworm and alopecia areata under one head is so important, that I will give Mr. Hutchinson's own concluding remarks, premising merely that I do not agree, by any means, with some of his views. His final remarks are rather long, but demand earnest attention.

Mr. Hutchinson's concluding remarks on the relation of Alopecia Areata to Ringworm :—

"Concluding Remarks."

"It will be seen that amongst the cases which I have related there are many in which the evidence was quite clear that ringworm had preceded the alopecia. There are also some in which no proof of such connection could be produced. There are several in which two members of the same family, who had suffered at the same time from ringworm, became subsequently the subjects of alopecia. In several instances the history of the original attack of ringworm was, in the first instance, denied by the patient, having been either not known or forgotten, but was subsequently supplied. The cases are a fair specimen of my personal experience during the last few years in reference to the disease in question, and their results will, I suspect, differ only from those of other observers in that, being specially interested in the point, I have been more patient than usual in seeking for the history of ringworm. Much patience is indeed necessary on the point, for I have found that almost invariably the first answer to the question. "Have you ever had ringworm when a child ?" is in a strong negative. Some patients have quite forgotten it ; some never knew what the disease was ; some doubted the diagnosis; and one and all are very willing, if they can, to ignore the fact. Inquiries on this head must be expected to give negative results in hospital practice far more frequently than amongst private patients. The later are more intelligent as to their antecedents, and can usually inquire at home as to what happened in their youth, with much better hope of success. I freely admit that in a very considerable number of cases, even after painstaking inquiry, no history of antecedent ringworm is forthcoming. These cases, however, do not shake my belief in the creed that alopecia areata is a disease in connection with cryptogamic growth. I suspect that some of them are examples of direct contagion from alopecia itself ; others of contagion to the heads of adults from ringworm in children ; and, lastly, others of contagion from pityriasis versicolor. Concerning the latter malady I have no doubt that it is transmutable with ringworm. My theory respecting alopecia is that is due to some from of cryptogamic life, which develope deeply in the hair fallicle, and does not grow in the hairs themselves. I admit that this cryptogam has not yet been satisfactorily identified by the microscope, and that in the majority of cases the most careful examination will fail to give any indication of its presence. Alopecia areata is, however a disease of such definite features, and of such remarkable sameness in its clinical history in different cases, that it is extremely difficult to entertain the belief that it depends on one cause

in one case, and upon a totally
different one in another. I cannot
but think that its cases ought all to
be placed in one group, and since
the evidence is so strong that some
of them depend on antecedent ringworm or upon direct contagion, I
cannot escape the conviction that
they all do so.

"There are certain other facts
which favour the belief just ex-
pressed. Thus, although alopecia
but rarely exhibits contagious properties, it sometimes does so. Many
authors have recorded instances in
which it affected several members
of the same family, and more than
one series of facts are on record in

which it prevailed as a household
epidemic.∗

"The entire absence of any form
of ill-health in the subjects of alopecia areata induced me to put
wholly aside any inquiry on that

∗ "By far the best example of epidemic
alopecia with which I am acquainted was
recorded in the *Boston Medical and Surgical
Journal,* May 1862. I am indebted to Dr.
Richmond Leigh for a detailed abstract of
this important paper. It occured in an
orphan asylum for girls, and no fewer than
sixty-one out of sixty-nine suffered. The
first case occured in January, the second in
March, and between the latter date and June
1st of the total of sixty-one had been completed.
The matron and four older girls who acted
as her assistants escaped. Dr. Bowen and
Dr. J. C. White both of Boston, and dis-
tinguished dermatologists, saw the cases, and
both agree that their general features were
indistinguishable from those of alopecia
areata and both failed, on microscopic
examination to direct the presence of any

score. We may, I think, entertain absolute incredulity as to what is called the neurotic form of this disease. It attacks young people

---

cryptogam. The hair-bulbs were wasted, as in alopecia. The bald patches are stated to have been smaller and more numerous. No preceding stage in the last resembling ringworm had been observed in any of the cases. Most of the cases were getting well in the course of a few months, and it was not thought that the cure was due to the use of any particular remedy. On this point, however, there is much room for fallacy.

"Whatever opinion we may incline to entertain as to the name which we should apply to the disease in this very remarkable outbreak, it appears to prove beyond dispute that there may occur a form of alopecia in patches which is actively contagious, and yet is unattended by any fungus which the most modern methods of research can demonstrate. The narrative may be placed side by side with those respecting certain other maladies, not usually virulently contagious, but which

more frequently than others, and
they are usually those in whom
neither headache nor any species
of neurotic disturbance had been
observed. It does not appear to
me to be worth while in such a
malady to ask an adult patient as
to overwork, mental worry, and the
like. Such influences may be found,
if sought for, in the majority of
those who consult us, and I feel
very certain that when they chance
to be coincident with alopecia they
do not stand to it in the relation of
the cause.

may by a sort of accident become so. I
allude to epidemics of pemphigoid porrigo,
such as those described in *Archives*, vol. iii.
p. 206, to those of puerperal fever, as related
by the late Mr. Storrs of Doncaster, and to
those of epidemic eczema in workhouses,
which have recently claimed much notice in
my pages."

"The mode in which alopecia develops, the frequent, or indeed usual, absence of bilateral symmetry, and of any definite unilateral asymmetry, the rounded form of its patches, and their tendency to enlarge serpiginously, are also, I think, conclusive evidence as to its not being of neurotic origin. We know of no neurotic malady which has round patches that spread at their edges.

"Lastly, I may allege that the modes of cure in alopecia areata by chrysophanic acid, creosote, blistering, etc., are all in favour of the belief that it is a disease of local origin. So also the facts that it always begins as a single patch, and, when it becomes general, spreads by the development of other patches from the parent as a centre, favour the belief in its cryptogamic nature. The facts as regards the occasional re-growth of hair, and, after an interval, its falling off again, are very curious. They are not susceptible of satisfactory explanation on any theory that I am acquainted with, but they fit more nearly with some facts that have been established as regards cryptogamic life than with any other hypothesis.

"Summary

"I may venture to offer the following conclusions as a summary of my present belief in reference to alopecia areata ;—

"*1st.* It is probable that all the cases which are well characterised, by abruptly rounded and quite smooth patches, are of one and the same nature as regards causation (possibly there is some slight exception to this in reference to syphilis).

"*2nd.* It is probable that all cases of well-characterised alopecia areata are in some connection, remote or direct, with the presence of a cryptogam.

"*3rd.* Many cases, probably the majority, occur in patients who have, at some former period, themselves suffered from ringworm.

"*4th.* A few cases occur to those who have never shown signs of ringworm, but who have, at some former period, been exposed to its contagion. Some cases occur to adults as the direct result of ringworm-contagion from children.

"*5th.* In a few cases it is possible that pityriasis versicolor on the chest of an adult may be the cause of alopecia areata on the scalp.

"*6th.* There are a few cases in which ringworm assumes, from the first, the features of alopecia areata. These may occur both in children and adults.

7th. Lastly, the explanation of the frequency with which alopecia areata begins on the back of the head is probably that it is caught by contagion from the backs of chairs and cushions, etc."

Eczema of External Ear and Meatus.

Miss Ethel S., 14 years of age, was brought to me on September 29, 1891, suffering from a skin affection showing itself as eczema of the outer ear and meatus, the surface of which was wetting, shiny, and in part scaly, and the discharge would at times dry up into scabs. She has very large tonsils ; her throat is swelled and irritable, and in the early morning she feels sick. Her father was formerly cured by me of eczema ; and hence the young lady was brought to me. She was cured in about six months, the remedies being *Med*. 1000, and *Bacill*. 1000 and *CC*.

This young lady's father's sister has also been cured by me of eczema, and her brother is now under my care for very severe eczema.

There is a tragic circumstance connected with my professional relationship with this socially important family, and it is this : Fifteen years ago I was treating a wee child of another branch of this family also for eczema that extended to the greater part of the poor mite's whole body. I explained to the parents that I regarded the eczema in questions as of a very pronouncedly constitutional nature, and that it was this constitutional disease that caused the truly terrible eczematous ooze, the skin being merely the medium of relief of the organism. Hence I gave my opinion that it would be dangerous to use local applications to the skin, lest the relatively fair general state of the patient should be impaired ; nearly all the glands were enlarged, and primarily so, and not merely from cutaneous irritation, to which conclusion I came from finding such hyper-trophied or indurated glands in parts where there was no active eczema.

What I am trying to say just amounts to this : My treatment was given up in contempt because I would not give any ointment or wash whatever, and the services of an eminent dermatologist were secured. Things went on very smoothly for a very few weeks, but the patient not long afterwards died "of weakness and exhaustion."

In my judgment she died of the practical application of the dermatologist's gross ignorance of dermatology : bedaubing and besmearing the skin with medicinal substances was the work of this probably well-meaning medical man ; but oh ! the shallow, shallow work !

Acute Universal Erythema and Chronic Rheumatoid Arthritis.

A maiden lady, 56 years of age, came to consult me on October 16,

1890, for pretty severe rheumatoid arthritis of three years' standing, affecting hands, feet, elbows, and knees. Although fifty-six years of age her menses are regular. She has just returned from Buxton, which, she thinks, did her a little good. Her hands are swelled a good deal, so that they are not of much use to her. She has strumous scars in neck. The pains are described as worst when she starts off, and worse in the evening, and worse on the East Coast than in London. Patient had been vaccinated three times. *Bacillinum C.* was given for a month.

November 25, 1890.—The improvement is very great indeed,— in fact, quite startling, for all the pain has gone and the swelling has sensibly diminished ; feet better ; can stand better ; and, moreover, she sleeps so much better.

To continue the same medicine.

December 5.—Patient hurries to me to show me the dreadful state of her skin, which is covered all over with acute erythema, rather papular. She describes the irritation as terrible in the heat . . . , and . . . . the rheumatism had gone.

January 1, 1891.—With very great difficulty I prevented this lady from putting something on "to cure" the erythema ; in fact, I did not quite succeed, and the case that seemed perfectly cured is not quite cured really, as the hands are stiff again and somewhat swelled.

℞ *Thuja occidentalis* **30**.

February 19, 1891.—The hands are not so well.

℞ *Psor* **30**, and a month later *Bacill. C.* finished the cure.

The point of greatest interest to me in this narration is the vicarious erythema.

I saw a middle-aged lady yesterday whose hands are swelled and much disfigured by rheumatoid arthritis. The lady's sister tells me that the late Sir Erasmus Wilson once cured the lady of eczema ; and we know well what the great Erasmus's "cures" were.

Rhinophyma.

Genuine severe rhynophyma is not a common disease. One case was under me last year, but patient only came two or three times ; the last time I saw him, both he and I were satisfied that the nose was somewhat smaller. Cases that stand, so to speak, midway between nasal dermatitis and rhinophyma are not so rare ; I cured two such cases in 1891, and both with our common antisycotics, principally *Thuja*, *Sabina* and *Cupressus*, all used in dynamic dose, and no local application whatever.

Eczema in a Child of Three.

On may 10th, 1888, a lady brought her three-year-old little

boy to me to be treated for eczema in the bends of the knees ; these regions were pretty badly affected, and the little man's cervical glands were considerably enlarged. As the eczema was most trying in the warmth of the bed, I gave *Syph. CC.* in very infrequent doses for a month.

June 7.—Much better, notably of the glands, but the eruption still itches in the warmth. *Acidum uricum* 6, ʒij., three drops in water night and morning.

August 1.—Nearly well, *Acidum hippuricum*, the same as the previous prescription.

This finished the cure.

Case of Eczema Glandis of Six Years' Duration.

An unmarried rufous gentleman, 32 years of age, came under my observation on may 18, 1887, for left-sided varicocele and eczema of the glans and of the sulcus of the penis ; the eruption had been there for six years. Patient was *puceau*. He informed me that he had formerly had eczema on his head. I first gave him *Clematis erecta* 1^x, five drops in water twice a day, but with no benefit. In June and July, for about five weeks he was under *Malandrinum 30*, with very great amelioration ; and thereafter, for about the same length of time, he had from me *Melitagrinum C.*

This cured the eczema, and patient ceased attending. At the end of the year patient said there was a very little of the eczema still in the sulcus, but he did not think it worth while being treated for it.

Case of Eczema,

A married lady, 30 years of age mother of two children, was brought to me by her husband on December 4 1891, with pretty severe eczema that had been bad during the past eight months, and being specially bad in the bends of arms and on the face, and worst of all around the mouth ; most destressing of an evening. Her lips are dry. cracked, "for ever peeling." Patient's condition was so bad, her

general state so debilitated, her
appearance so old, worn, and weary,
that I felt it to be imperative to
better her blood life and pull her
together, so to speak, before setting
about a scientific cure of the case,
so I put her on *Levico* θ for a
few weeks, and then upon *Bellis
perennis* θ for a month, when patient would not come any more,
even to please her husband, remarking, "oh! I'm getting on nicely
now ; I do not want the doctor."

Case of Ringworm, Eczema, Acne, and Asthma.

A powerful, somewat asthmatic
gentleman, 58 years of age, came
from the north to consult me on
the 12th August 1891, telling me a

history of slight winter asthma for many years ; this he keeps down with Turkish baths, which he was taken regularly ever since he was 21 years of age. His appearance on being undressed was as if he had small-pox of moderate severity, only the pustules are those of acne. He tells me he had "three ring-worms across the belly" in the month of February 1881, which he got cured with ointments; and then he got eczema, and got this also cured with ointments ; and then came this pustular eruption which ointments will not cure.

℞ *Bacill.* 1000.

August 26.—Much better.

Rep.

September 8.—"Those powders are too much for me ; they cause me bad breathing and sickly feeling ; worse in the morning ; the skin is rather better ; there is no matter in it now."

He is much afraid of the powders, "they acts so powerfully."

October 2.—The skin is cleaning.

R *Rep.* (*CC.*)

Otober 16. Much better.

Rep. (C.)

October 30.—The chronic difficulty of breathing (the asthma) has gone, the breathing being now normal.

The same remedy was repeated a few times, and *Thuja* 30 was interpolated, when patient was well, and went abroad to divert his mind from grief due to the death of his wife.

The last time I saw him his exclamation was, I am so much bettr in myself,—infinitely better in every way."

Brawny Dermatitis.

An elderly gentleman consulted me on Nov. 12, 1890, for an eruption of the skin, that I can only call brawny dermatitis. It was all over his body, and had been there for years, and itches a great deal. This gentleman was discharged cured in less than a year, and still continues well. The remedies I used were *Persicaria urens* **30** and

3 *Urtica urens* θ, and *Sodium salicylate*.

Patient formerly suffered from chronic rheumatism, but ceased to do so after this rash came out.

Now he has neither skin disease nor rheumatism.

Very Severe Case of Sycosis.

On September 26, 1890, a London professional man, 41 years of age, married, and in fair general health, came to me as a *dernier ressort*, and on the earnest solicitation of a friend and neighbour. Said he : "I have always ridiculed homoeopathy, and do not believe in it the least little bit, but I am in despair ; I have had this beastly skin disease for twelve years (pointing to his chin and face), and I have been under treatment all the time by the most eminent surgeons of London ; altogether I have been under eleven different doctors,—of course all allopaths."

Patient's chin and face co-extensive with his beard, was a "mass of corruption,"—*i. e.*, dried up, caked together mattery ooze, which he was obliged to get off very frequently with the aid of poultice, when the surface was red and angry and shiny, the sticky stuff at once beginning to appear again. An ointment he uses keeps it down pretty well in the summer months, but is powerless from autumn to spring. He has also very severe pyorrhoea alveolaris ; his gums have receded, and

the bulk of his very beautifully
formed teeth have already fallen out
entire, or stand out from the gums
ready to fall out ; his breath is star-
coraceous, and his gums and mouth
generally he described as "rotten."
He has had recurrent opthalmia
many times. He tells me he has
used scores of ointments, and been
very severely handled by the skin
specialists, having undergone scari-
fications and epilations at many different times. Patient has been twice
vaccinated. The feeling in the diseased part he describes as stinging.
My treatment was continued till
June 10, 1892, when I was able to
declare him as he declared himself,
well.* Treatment extending over all

July 1893—Continues quite well.

these months necessarily comprises a number of remedies, the case being so severe and of such long standing. Practically patient had all the leading nosodic and other antisycotics. as well as *Zincum acet.* 1, *Jequirity 3ˣ*, *Levico* θ, (the strong water), *Chelidon majus* θ, and *Calc. sulph.*

Note on Levico.

The waters of *Levico* are a very favourite remedy of mine in many skin affections where I need a little tonic, and where it seems of great advantage to give the organism a rest from the effects of high dilutions of the more specifically acting remedies.

In very difficult and pathologically complicated cases the organism, under the influence of very high dilutions, appears to get excited and into a state of unrest; here progress seems suspended, and one then needs, figuratively speaking, a harmless material—something to clean the slate and so get a fresh start: this the strong water of *Levico* does beautifully. A capital way to administer it is to order ten drops in a wineglassful of warm water two or three times a day, by preference immediately after meals.

Offensive Perspirations—
Periodical Headaches.

An unmarried lady, 38 years of age, came under my care on

July 11, 1892, principally for *headaches* and *offensive perspirations*. Patient had lived some years in India, where she had ague badly. The headache was really brow-ague at a spot over the right eye, very bad at 7 P. M., and recurring every eleven days. The perspirations were described as *sour, oniony, nettly*.

℞ *Trit. 6 Nat. mur..* Six grains three times a day.

August 9.—The powders brought back the ague, of which patient had long been free ! Thereupon she immediately took quinine. Perspiration less offensive.

℞ *Nat. mur. 30.*

September 12.—Quite free from headaches, and the perspiration has ceased to be offensive. The cure had held good when I last saw patient in February 1893.

Lichen Urticarius.

A bonny boy, 2 ½ years of age, was brought by his mother to me on the 7th of August 1890 for lichen urticarius. But there was an even more distressing feature in this case, for this mite of a boy was already an inveterate masturbator. The urticarious spots were usually at their worst when he got warm in bed, or hot at any time. He had seatworms, picking his nose a good deal. He was about a year under my treatment, and was then discharged quite cured, not only of his cutaneous affection, but also of his nose-

picking and of his secret habit of
mauling himself about; for it was
noteworthy that while he would
pick his nose freely enough before
folks, and even notwithstanding
their forbidding it, he did not mas-
turbate other than in secret.

The remedy that cured the skin
affection was very evidently *Bacillinum C.* during one month at the
beginning of the cure, and the
same remedy in the two-hundredth
dilution later on. The remedy that
cured his secret habit was very
clearly *Platina 30*, under which he
was during three separate (not con-
secutive) months. There were inter-
current ailings—cough, cold, an-
orexia—and *Thuja 30*, *Ipec. 1*,
Ledum 3ˣ, and *Med. CC.* respec-

tively came into play. The precise parts played by these other four remedies in this case I could not quite determine. More particularly, I do not know which cured the seatworms. But, as before stated, I am very sure the lichen was cured by the *Bacill.*, and the masturbation was cured by the *Platina 30.*

[On the subject of *Platina* in this regard, see Grauvogl's *Lehrbuch.*]

Remarks on the Origin of Self-Abuse In Children.

The case of lichen urticarious just related teaches a lesson which physicians and parents might with advantage remember. We are far too apt to suppose that vice and vicious habits are due to abstract sin trickling down upon us from the dim and distant past, or as simply generated, as it were, afresh by innate sinfulness. Well, in this we err egregiously. The best way to get at the core of a nebulous subject is to take concrete cases separately, from the very simplest standpoint. So let us take this simple case of nettle-rash. What was the nature of the lichen? Was it morally sinful?

Clearly it was simply physical disease, and in this case probably from the boy's father. Was the nose-picking a sinful habit? or due to physical disease? By common consent nose-picking indicates gastric irritation, and most frequently worms gets the blame. This boy had worms.

We do not reckon his lichen or his worms unto him as sin, but recognize their simple morbid basis, and use remedies to cure them.

So I do with masturbation generally ; so I did with this boy's secret habit, that, left uncured, would most probably have resulted in his becoming both physically and morally a wreck. But not only was the secret habit in this child completely cured, but he, in the words of his mother, "does not like to do so,"— *i. e.*, his sweeter (*healthy*) moral self shrinks from the very idea.

Have the schools any therapeusis
to compare to this ? I suppose a
soothing lotion or ointment for the
child's moral nature.

Eczema of Ears of Seven Years' Standing.

On August 20, 1887, a little girl
of nine was brought to me for an
ill-smelling discharge from the
ears, that was said to have started
after she had had dysentery seven
years previously. In the fold of the
left arm a little eczema. Although
only nine years old the child had
been twice vaccinated, and was
clearly quite blighted thereby.

After being under treatment by
Thuja occidentalis **30** for a month,

my note runs, "Vast improvement all round."

After a few weeks respectively of *Sabina* **30** and *Sulphur* **30**, patient left cured at the end of the year 1887.

Flat Papilloma in the Anal Region

A childless married lady, a little over **30** years of age, came under my observation on July 19, 1887, for certain very distressing symptoms in the anal region, preventing sleep at night : worse at 2 A. M. On examining the parts I found the anal opening surrounded by haemorrhoidal buttons, and on the tip of one of these a flat papil-

loma about the size of a split horse-
bean. By day the whole region
was exceedingly uncomfortable
only, but by night its soreness
prevented sleep.

℞ *Syp. CC.*

August 16.—Very much better
indeed ; sleeps now quite well.
An examination shows that the
papilloma has quite disappeared.

Patient remained another
couple of weeks under my treatment for the haemorrhoids. These
quite disappeared during that
period under the influence of, first,
Spiritus glandium quercus θ, and then
of *Euphorbia amygdaloides.*

Pruritus Ani.

A general staff-officer, no longer young, came under my care on Dec. 11, 1891, complaining bitterly of being roused up at night with fearful itching at the anus. An examination of the part showed only the very slightest degree of eczema. Being of opinion that the pruritus was due to port wine, I ordered *Spiritus glandium quercus*, ten drops in water night and morning. This cured the pruritus. When I next saw the general he said, "That's all right; now I want something for my bronchitis." The complaint was chronic winter catarrh of the bronchial lining. The *Acetum Lobeliæ*, in four-drop

doses every four hours, quite cured
this in about three weeks.

Case of Bat's Wing Disease—
Lupus.

A maiden lady, 48 years of age,
from Shropshire, came on August
5th. 1892, to consult me for an eruption on her nose and two cheeks,
the figure thus produced being
responsible for the designation of
bat's-wing disease. The eruption
is getting very, very slowly worse
for the past twelve years. The skin
peels off in little flakes, leaving the
underlying skin red, and this again
dries and in its turn peels off, but
very, very slowly and the whole of
the skin is not involved, there being
healthy skin between. Patient's

father is stated to have died of decline at 57 years of age, and her mother, patient tells me, died at 52 of mesenteric atrophy. One of patien'ts brothers died of phthisis, and her other six brothers all died in infancy. Her three sisters are alive. Patient has had active treatment, principally *Arsenic* and *Mercury.*

℞ *Bacill.* **CC.**

September 2.—The bat's wing is half gone !

℞ *Rep.*

Sept. 30.—Nose quite free, except in the right side near the eye, where it is *more active.*

Patient informs me that she has been three times vaccinated.

℞ *Thuja 30.*

Nov. 4.—There is just one small spot of the eruption left, near the corner of the eye. A good deal of haemorrhage from the rectum.

℞ *Bacill. CC.*

December 9.—Patient writes me under this date from her home: "I have *no trace of the disease left*, but the piles have bled on four occasions. I was so well while taking the powder."

℞ *Rep.*

January 13, 1893.—The skin remains quite well. "I eat double."

And four months later the lady's sister, in answer to my inquiry, informed me that patient continued perfectly well.

Papular Rash.

An unmarried lady, 23 years of age, was brought to me by her elder sister on Dec. 15, 1890, for a very disagreeable rash on the body. The patient had had measles, whooping-cough, chicken-pox, and jaundice during the course of her little life, and had also been twice vaccinated. Her menses were irregular; she suffered from nose-bleed. The eruption occupied the skin over the chest, stomach, and duodenum, and itched a good deal on going to bed. Patient is very costive, anaemic, and complains pretty eloquently of flatulent dyspepsia. Her spleen is enlarged; she twitches and jumps (starts) a good deal; is better in the evening, worse in the morning.

℞ *Thuja occidentalis* **30**, in infrequent doses.

In two months patient had gained five pounds in weight and was quite well, barring an enlarged spleen and little spells of nose-bleed. This was cured in a few weeks by *Urtica urens* θ, ten drops in water at bed time, and the young lady has continued to thrive ever since, so her mother told me quite lately.

I have often maintained the reality of voccinosis as a morbid entity, and as the years roll round I become more and more certain of my thesis. See my little treatise "On Vaccinosis."

Epidemic Eczema.

The only epidemic of eczema, apparently contagious, within my experience was one that broken out in the spring of 1891 at a very large public school near London.

The news came to me thus :—

March 16, 1891."

"Dear Sir.—On or about the 5th of this month a spot appeared over the eyebrow of the bearer (my son). Thinking it merely a bruise received the previous day whilst playing football, a piece of gum paper was put over the place.

"A few days served to show that the thing was more than a simple bruise, so we sent him over to Dr. ——, of—— ; he also thought it merely an unhealthy wound, ordered on a bread poultice, and gave some ointment to be applied when 'the wound' was cleaned. At the end of two days I felt sure the diagnosis had been wrong, and so sent the boy over again to the doctor. It was then pronounced to be eczema.

"*Rhus tox.* inwardly, and zinc ointment externally, were prescribed and a fish, fruit. and vegetable diet insisted upon.

"This morning the thing has assumed such alarming proportions that my husband and I felt we must have your advise regarding it.

"Three of the boys playing in his team have broken out with the same kind of eruption."

There were quite a number of cases besides these, patient's brother being one of them.

The eruption itched very much in the evening, and had spread a good deal when the lad called upon me with the just-cited letter of his mother.

The iodide of sulphur in the third trituration, and six-grain doses frequently repeated, cured the eczema in both lads in about six weeks, and there has not been any return of it.

THE CONSTITUTIONAL CURE OF ALOPECIA AREATA.

The Direct Art Cure of Spotbaldness, or Alopecia Areata, by Internal Medication.

BARRING a certain number of homoeopathic physicians, the universal treatment of spot-baldness is by local measures, and one never hears of any constitutional cure. And yet such a state of one's scalp can hardly be health. Jonathan Hutchinson, who has vast experience, says : "The entire absence of

any form of ill-health in the subjects of alopecia areata induces me
to put wholly aside any inquiry on
that score (*i. e.*, ill-health)."

Hutchinson also believes that
pityriasis versicolor "is transmutable with ringworm." We thus have
three name-having ailments, viz.—
ringworm, pityriasis versicolor, and
alopecia areata, that are not accompanied by any ill-health at all; such
are the views held, but they are not
mine, inasmuch as I am unable to
believe such things, and my experience contradicts them.

Of ringworm, I have already
treated in a separate (already referred to) Monograph; with alopecia
areata we are here concerned. I

have examined a goodly number of cases of ringworm, and never yet found a really healthy individual suffering therefrom : certainly they were not ill in bed or ill in themselves at the time, but a constitutional taint I could discover in almost every case, *i. e.*, a phthisical taint, near or remote.

I find the same taint in alopecia areata, but often another taint also. A word or two on the function of the hair may not be amiss.

Exner has published, in a recent number of the *Wiener Klinische Wochenschrift*, an article on this interesting subject. He states at the outset that the disposition of the hair on the different parts of the body always serves a definite object. The study of the descent of man and of embryology has shown that our ancestors were entirely covered with hair, as are the anthropoid apes. According to Darwin, the gradual disappearance of the hair is due to the repulsion felt by women for hairy men, and their liking for the opposite ; that is, to sexual selection. In the same manner he explains the exaggerated development of the hairy scalp in women, and of the beard in men, for in women the long hair and in men the beard have always been considered as attributes of beauty.

As to the physiologic functions of hairs, it is admitted that they are modified sense-organs, which have lost some of their connections with the nerves. It is probable that in primitive man the distribution of the hair upon the body was irregular, and that the length, colour, structure and thickness of the hair varied with functions for which it was intended. The hair which has been left upon the body in the process of evolution has been left there for a definite purpose. Certain hairs serve as organs of touch ; notably the eyelashes, the bulbs of which are surrounded by a network of nerve fibres, and in a less degree the hairs of the eyebrows. Both these serve to protect the eyes ; for being sensitive, they give warning of danger, so that reflex closure of the lids is produced. The eyebrows also prevent drops of sweat from running into the eyes, while the eyelashes keep out dust. The eyebrows and lashes also serve a purpose in sexual selection. The down which covers the body is also endowed with tactile sense ; the hair in the region of the genitals and anus being the least sensitive. A thick growth of hair is also found in those parts of the body where friction must take place between contiguous cutaneous surfaces, as in the axillae, groin, perineo-scrotal and perineo-vulvar regions. By experiment with pieces of skin covered with hair, Exner has shown that the hairy covering markedly diminishes the friction of the cutaneous surfaces.

In animals the hair serves to maintain and regulate the heat of the body, but in man the hair of the scalp alone serves this purpose. Hair is itself a poor conductor of heat, and retains air, also a poor conductor in its interstices.

The fact that the forehead is not covered with hair, Exner explains on the theory that in the contest between the natural tendency of the hair to protect the head against changes of temperature and the tendency of human nature towards beauty, the latter has prevailed more easily because the non-conducting properties of that portion of the skull are increased by the air containing frontal sinuses, and that that portion of the head is easily protected from the heat of the sun by inclining the head forward.

What is the nature of Alopecia Areata?

In as much as opinions are so much divided on the true nature of this peculiarly interesting affection, I have thought that it might be settled clinically.

Is it related to ringworm, or not?

Now ringworm is very obviously accompanied by fungi—always, they say. Nobody can find any fungi in alopecia areata, still they may be present for all that, though they have not been found.

Is Alopecia Areata catching ?

The question, according to Hutchinson, must be answered in the affirmative; according to Alder Smith, on the other hand, it must be answered in the negative—the former is a high authority, but so is the latter. Hutchinson even explains its favourite habitat at the back of the head, as due to the infection coming from the backs of chairs and from cushions.

Both Hutchinson and Alder Smith are original observers, and from their opinions on the facts given by their own observations. My own experience goes to show that alopecia areata is *not* catching —that is, I have never been able to trace a case of such alopecia either from or to another person.

Now what clinical evidence have I which goes to show that alopecia areata can be cured by the internal administration of remedies ? and, this given, how does the same shed light upon the nature of the cases ? Let me begin with a brief narration of a case which, seen in the light of much previous experience as to phthisis, ringworm, and vaccinosis, indicates its double nature :—

Alopecia Areata.

A married gentleman, 34 years of age, came under my observation in the month of April 1894 ; circular baldness in patches here and there, also both ends of moustache are gone; much indigestion and phlegm for many years, and these symptoms led me to prescribe *Thuja 30* ; and when he returned after a month of this remedy he complained of the violent action of the *Thuja 30*. "Those powders have so upset me that I have had to keep my bed."

No medicine.

July 17.—Mending very beautifully, but quite lately the hair is falling out again very badly.

No medicine.

Aug. 20.—℞ Bacill. *30*.

Oct. 23.—Hair growing everywhere very well.

℞ *Rep.*

He called a year later with catarrhal symptoms of chest.

℞ *Rep.*

And twice subsequently the same remedy was repeated. Discharged quite cured in the fall of 1896.

Alopecia Areata in a Lady of 35 Years of Age.

A married lady, 35 years of age, mother of three children, was brought by her husband to see me in the spring of 1897, for certain nerve symptoms, and, . . . "I have a bald patch on my head, about the size of a shilling, also two small wens on the left side of my head, in the hair."

April 1.—Bacill. *30.*

May 4.—Wens gone; urine very thick. *Tub. test* C.

June 1.—"I am much better ; the scurf in my hair is very troublesome, but I believe the hair is growing on the little bald patch which I showed you."

June 29.—Not quite so well ; very scurfy scalp.

℞ *Tub. test. C.*

July. 27.—Bacill. **C.**

We had here arrived at a point where further progress seemed barred.

Aug. 26.—℞ *Thuja occid. 30.*

Sept. 23.—"I have been to my hair-dresser's, and he tells me I have not nearly so much scurf on my head, and the bald patch is quite covered with hair."

Loss of Moustache.

A staff-officer, 59 years of age, came under my observation in 1894, first for debility, that remained after influenza. After being under *Urtica ur.* and *Cypripedium pub.* θ for six weeks, he was practically well; "but," said he, "look at the left side of my moustache; the hair is all coming out, and in places the hair of my head. I can't sleep."

April 2.—℞ *Bacill. 30.*

June 11.—Some vomiting; sleepless broken; the hair is visibly thicker, the roundish patch no longer so evidently circular,

℞ *Rep.*

Aug. 15.—Nearly well, moustache much thicker.

℞ *Rep.*

Oct. 24, 1898.—Well; moustache flourishing

This case is interesting, because only one remedy was used all the time (infrequent doses), and the influence of this upon the hair-growth was quite evident. At the beginning of the treatment the moustache had almost gone on the left side, and at about the centre of this left side it was practically hairless, and even on the right side the rest while well-grown moustache was indeed a sorry thing. It is more than two years since patient

was discharged cured, and the cure
holds good to date. Said I the
other day to his daughter, "How's
your father's moustache ?"

"Oh ! it's all right ; as good as
ever, but much more grey ; poor
dear papa, he *was* in a way about
his moustache."

Case of Alopecia Areata.

A very tall lad, fifteen years of
age, came under my observation in
March 1893, to be treated for alopecia areata of moderate severity.
"Large bald patches." There were
scars in the right side of the neck,
where glands had seemingly been
excised ; some not very large indurated glands in both sides of the
neck and in both groins. The young

man's skin almost literally covered with severe acne. "A mass of pustules" is the note in my book—the patches had not the dry, clean, ivorylike surface we are accustomed to see in alopecia areata, but they were sticky and shiny, and he scratched them a good deal. This led me to *Mal. C.*, and a seemingly perfect cure resulted in three months. And eighteen months later a lady friend of patient's family said to me, "You made a wonderful cure of General X——'s son's head."

In April 1895 the young man turned up again, but this time with only one bald patch over his left ear, "size of a crown piece."

℞ *Mal. C.*

May 2.—Patch smaller, and hair growing on it.—*Rep.*

June 6.—No further progress. ℞ *Bacill. 30.*

July 16.—Hair growing ; neck-glands going down.—*Rep.*

Sept.—Well.

Two years later. His cousin informs me that the cure holds good.

Alopecia Areata.

The Countess, X——, aet. 50, mother of a family, came under my observation for bald circular patches at the back of her head, that have been there only a short time she thinks, and for which she has been under eminent specialists, who say it is a nerve affection. Her ladyship has a marvellous head of hair particularly for one of her age, and hence it would seem almost more strange that she should have perfectly bald circular patches in amongst such a mass of hair, strong and long reaching, a little armful in quantity, down to her hips. But so it was.

Four or five months under *Bacillinum* resulted in a perfect cure ; the patches lost their shiny aspect and slowly covered with little hairs, and in about six months it was impossible to find them. The cure holds good to date.

Most of the cases of alopecia areata that have come under my care have been persons naturally blessed with uncommonly fine heads of hair.

Severe Case.

Lady X——, married, childless, 41 years of age, came under me in April 1896. She wore a wig, and had numerous typical bald areas all over the scalp, and what little of the scalp was not affected by the alopecia, the hair thereon was cropped as stubble. She had tried so many things, and so many physicians, surgeons, and hair professors, that she had quite given up all idea of ever being any better— had indeed become quite callous about it, and did not as a matter of fact consult me about her alopecia at all, but about recurrent cysts ;

and it was only by accident that I discovered the alopecia one day when the wig was off, because of the great heat.

The case concerns us here only for the alopecia areata, and as very many constitutional remedies were used, I am not able to say what remedies cured, but in less than a year, the alopecia was quite cured, and a year after beginning the treatment the wig could be entirely discarded, but the new hair was not yet long enough for her to dispense with some artificial hair arrangement at the back.

"All my life," she gave as the duration of her alopecia ; so a complete cure with remedies within a year is not bad. *Thuja* **30.** *Bacill.* **30.** *Sul.* **30.** *Psor.* **C.** *Hydrastis* θ, and *Urtica* θ, were amongst the remedies used, and that they, or some of them, cured, admits of no doubt whatever, as no local application whatever was ordered by me, and the case had gone on for so many many years, inspite of the best and the worst treatment known in this London.

INDEX.

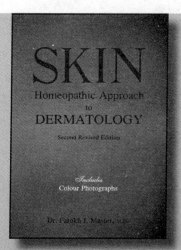

Skin – Homeopathic Approach to Dermatology
(Second Revised Edition)

Farokh J. Master

- Covers wide array of information on skin disorders
- Coloured photographs, description of home remedies and the homeopathic approach are some of its highlighting features
- Completely re-written in light of the present day knowledge

ISBN: 978-81-319-0716-0 | 1036pp | HB

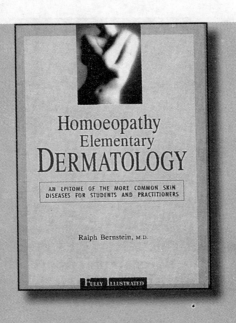

Homeopathy Elementary Dermatology

Bernstein Ralph

Illustrations (An Epitome of the More Common Skin Diseases for Students & Practitioners)

ISBN: 81-8056-389-8 Book Code BB5733 | 326pp | PB

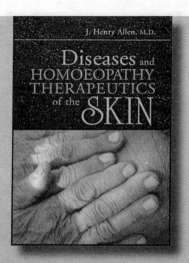

Diseases and Homoeopathy Therapeutics of the Skin

J. Henry Allen, M.D.

- Description, etiology, diagnosis and treatment of various skin diseases according to the law of similars
- The history, pathology and anatomy of skin has been described briefly
- Dermatological therapeutics has been elaborated beautifully

ISBN: 978-81-319-0018-5 | BA–2007 | 344pp | PB

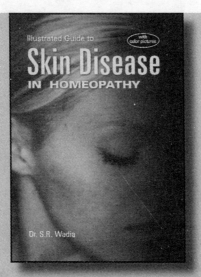

Illustrated Guide to Skin Disease in Homeopathy

Dr S. R. Wadia

- The book is a handy reference guide which illustrates the scope of homeopathy in dermatology
- It would help the practitioner to decide which cases he can treat and how

ISBN : 978-81-319-0177-9 | 72pp | PB

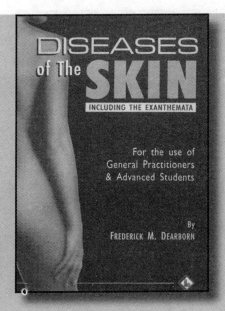

Diseases of the Skin

Dearborn F.M.

For the use of General Practitioners & Advanced Studies
for Students (with illustrations)

ISBN: 81-7021-230-8 | Book Code: BD 2187
570pp | PB

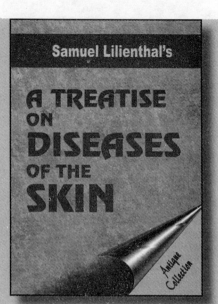

A Treatise on Diseases
of the Skin

Lilienthal S.

An Antique Collection

**ISBN: 81-8056-076-7 | BL5659
272pp | PB**

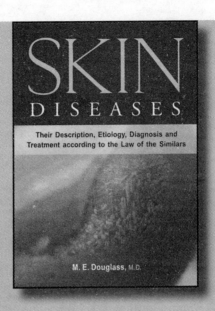

Skin Diseases

Douglas M.E.

Their Description, Etiology, Diagnosis & Treatment According to the Law of the Similars

ISBN: 81-7021-316-9 | Book Code BD 2194
456pp | PB

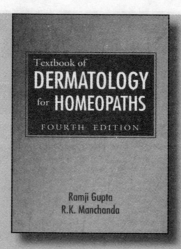

Textbook of Dermatology for Homeopaths

Ramji Gupta & R.K. Manchanda

- Improved edition with more than 200 coloured clinical photographs, which help to illustrate the text

- Suggests specific homeopathic remedies for every disease along with general instructions for their management

- Covers wide array of information on skin diseases including hereditary disorders, naevi, metabolic disorders, leprosy, viral infections etc.